MELISSA RYAN

STRENGTH TRAINING FOR WOMEN

Empower Your Body, Empower Your Life
(2024 Guide for Beginners)

Copyright © 2023 by Melissa Ryan

All rights reserved. No part of this publication may be reproduced, stored or transmitted in any form or by any means, electronic, mechanical, photocopying, recording, scanning, or otherwise without written permission from the publisher. It is illegal to copy this book, post it to a website, or distribute it by any other means without permission.

First edition

This book was professionally typeset on Reedsy.
Find out more at reedsy.com

Contents

1	Strength Training and Yoga for Beginners	1
2	Home Exercises	4
3	Foods to Consume	24
4	Healthy Recipes	28
5	Tips for Novices	48
6	Beginning Yoga	53
7	Yoga Program	60
8	Yoga Training Schedule	69
9	Suggestions for Novices	77

1

Strength Training and Yoga for Beginners

Why Women Should Engage in Strength Training

Most people assume strength training is a sport best left to men. Because they were afraid of coming out as "overly masculine," women would frequently look down on the bodybuilding idea. Alternatively, a lot of women prefer to dedicate a significant amount of time to various forms of training, such cardio and light toning. Your body can never really change its shape unless you begin strength training, even while these workouts can help you lose body fat and tone your muscles to some extent.

Losing Weight with Strength Training

Gaining that "hourglass shape" and reducing body fat are goals shared by all women. Cardio and core-strengthening exercises are essential if you wish to have this amazing body. A more defined upper body can be achieved by strength training, which will increase the muscle in your back and shoulders. Enhance my writing style by adding flare to my lower body. Strength training also helps draw attention to my legs and hips. Building strength in your biceps and triceps can assist address the issue of flabby arms, which is a complaint often voiced by women.

Your body will burn fat and calories even with a basic strength exercise program. Strengthening your body with resistance training exercises is the goal of lifting weights. Your metabolism is raised by this kind of workout, which also replaces fat with muscle. The rise in your resting metabolic rate causes your body to start burning calories even when you're not moving. Regarding weight loss, this is quite beneficial. Eating more calories and chipping away at the fat deposits that have been bothering you during previous workout regimens are necessary for building muscle. You'll get stronger and leaner after strength training.

Strength Training for Wellness Purposes

The risk of osteoporosis can be decreased, which is just one of the advantages of strength training for women. You may strengthen your bones in addition to your muscles through weight training. You have a lower chance of fractures and shattered bones since it promotes bone density. Stronger and healthier spines can be achieved by weight training, according to research that suggests it can boost spinal bone density.

In addition to lowering back pain, strength training helps with posture. You can develop a taller physique with a straight spine, shoulders, and back by strengthening your core, back, and shoulders with weight training. It also helps to address improper posture. Lower back discomfort is also avoided with this.

Lifting weights improves your mood and lowers stress. Exercise and weight lifting cause endorphins to be released. Neurotransmitters known as endorphins combat sadness, stop pain, and elevate mood. Due to mental stimulation, an increase in endorphins also increases energy and enhances attentiveness.

Working Out to Get Stronger

Strength training can help you perform everyday chores like lifting or moving objects much more easily. It can also help you stay injury-free and gain more stamina. Maybe your fear of looking like the Incredible Hulk has kept you from starting strength training. Fear not. Because men's and women's hormones function differently, guys experience all of that mass more frequently. It is true that women cannot develop the massive biceps that men bodybuilders have, even though they may lift more weights on a daily basis and increase their dosage. You'll appear sleek and muscular, yet incredibly feminine, instead. Become aware of every muscle in your body to build a robust, well-rounded body.

Should you be debating whether to begin lifting weights, you should give strength training a serious thought because it has so many amazing benefits for ladies. You will quickly start to look and feel better if you do the at-home strength training exercises in this book.

2

Home Exercises

Home Exercises for Strengthening

As a novice, you might feel better at ease working out at home, even though many bodybuilders love coming to the gym. No expensive equipment or specialized gym is needed for the many fantastic weightlifting exercises that you can perform in the comfort of your own home. Try these at-home strength training exercises to get a sense of the types of movements and lifting you'll need to do to build strength.

Exercises for Warming Up

When you start a strength training program, it's crucial to warm up since it tells your body and mind that you will soon be engaging in some physical action. These are some crucial steps in preparing your body for higher-intensity workouts.

Cardio

Warm up your body with moderate exercise for 15 to 20 minutes at first. Your heart rate will rise as a result, your metabolism will speed up, and your muscles will become loose and heated. The cardio option that appeals to you the most should be the one you choose for your warm-up. There are various possibilities available. The recommended activity is a vigorous ten-minute walk, but if you'd like to speed up the pace, you can also jog or even sprint. Go for a bike ride, jump rope, do some Zumba, or perform cardiovascular exercises. Prior to beginning the actual workout with weights, the objective is to increase your heart rate and get your body moving.

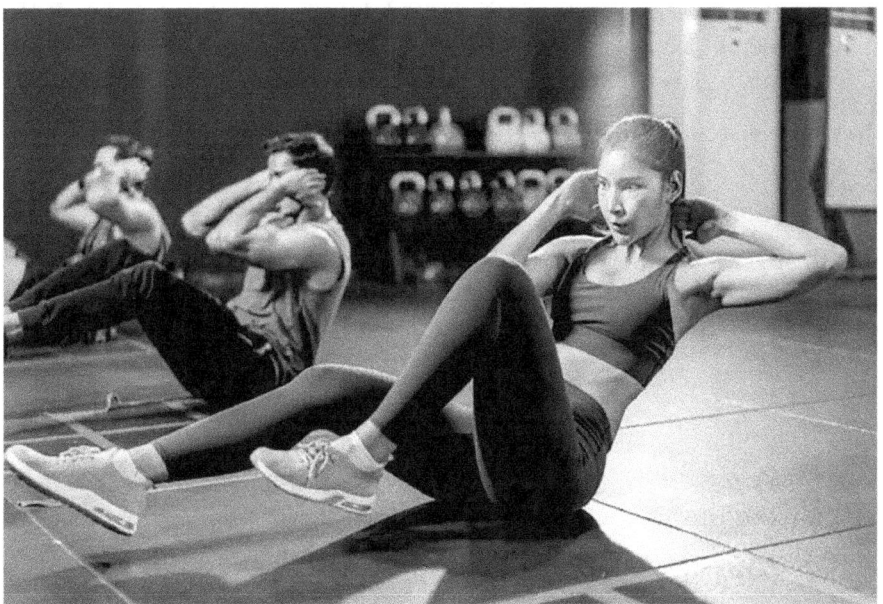

Adaptive Extending

Being somewhat adaptable will help a lot. You will notice an improvement in your range of motion and a greater sense of flexibility as you continue to tone your body. Your flexibility will improve and you'll get closer to your strength goals if you stretch before and after your exercises.

1. To begin, perform a few simple toe touches. Stretching your arms above your head, take a standing position with your feet together and bend the waist slowly. Even though your rear legs will start to pull, keep lowering yourself

toward the ground. Try reaching your fingertip tips toward your toes. It's okay if the initial attempt doesn't get you that far. With continued effort, you'll grow closer and closer. Reposition yourself to a standing position after a brief period of time. Five times over, repeat this.

2. Proceed to perform Linear Marches and Skips after that. Just lift your knee to your waist and lower your foot back to the ground to complete the basic marching motion. On the other foot, repeat. Stepping back and forth, march through your room three times. Afterwards, transition it into a skip, when you leap while kicking up your knee and walking. Keep your knees up to your waist as you skip three times around the room.

3. Next comes warming up the upper body. Make sure your feet are shoulder-width apart as you perform some Arm Circles. When you raise both arms together and swing them in a full circle, begin with your hands by your sides. Perform 10 sets of swings, 10 forward swings and 10 backward swings.

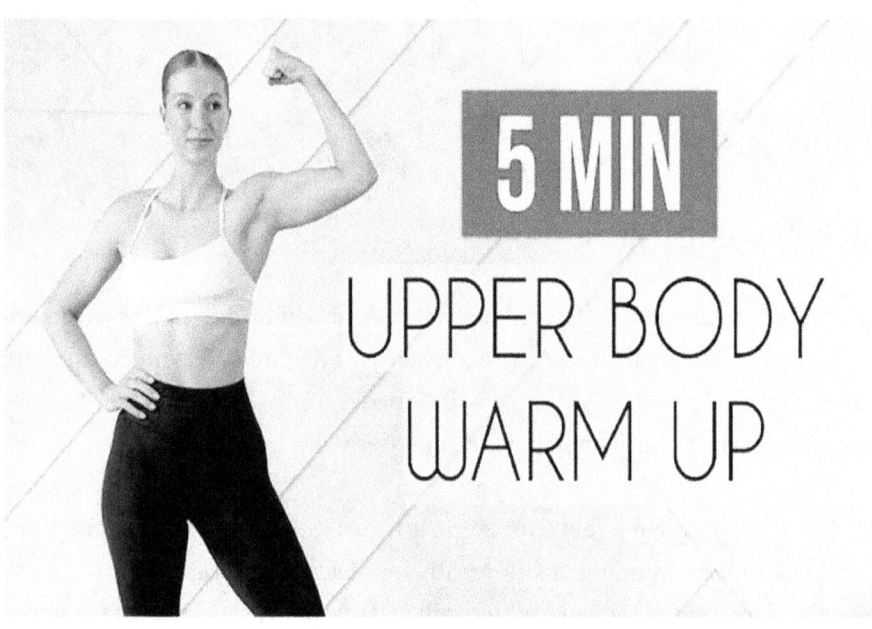

HOME EXERCISES

Fairness

Bodybuilding relies heavily on balance, thus one of the things you should practice throughout your warm-up is learning how to maintain your focus while balanced.

1. Prior to dead lifting, warm up. Arms by your sides and feet together, take a stance. Return to the starting position by raising your right arm and left leg simultaneously. Perform ten repetitions of this, then switch to raise your left arm and leg. Do ten repetitions of those as well.

2. Take a duck walk. Maintain a straight back as you crouch and begin walking gently, never rising to a standing posture but always keeping your back straight as you descend. Repeat these three steps around your room.

3. Pack some yoga mats. Lift your arms above your head and stand with your legs together. Ten seconds should pass while you raise and extend your right leg in front of your torso. After lowering it, extend your left leg and repeat the action. Perform five leg raises.

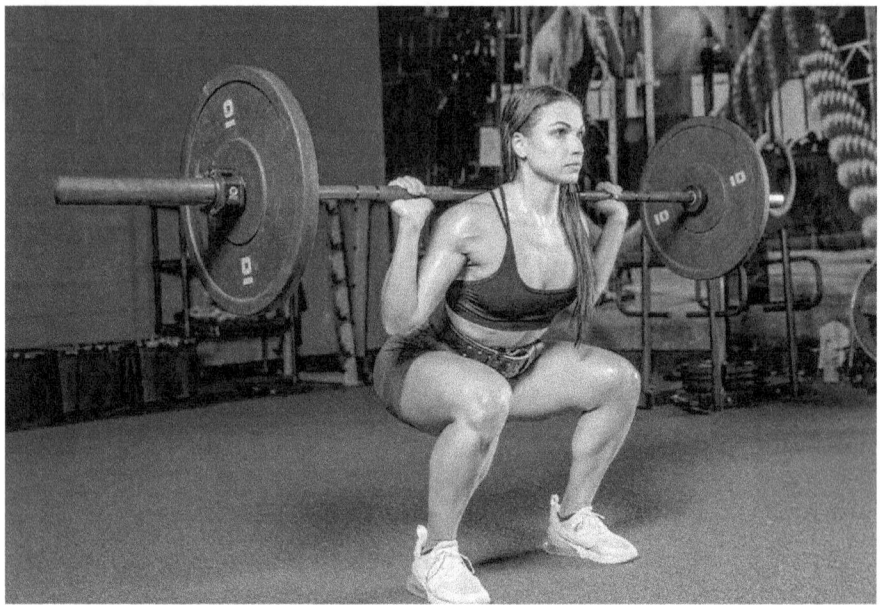

Upper Body Exercises

The back, shoulders, chest, and arms are the main areas to concentrate on when building your upper body. You can achieve a stronger upper body by mastering these exercises, which are simple enough even for novices. Simply pushing and pulling is how the upper body is worked. Two portions comprise these exercises.

Do three sets of twelve dumbbell curls on each side when pulling

1. Dumbbell weights should be chosen so that you can begin comfortably. Three, five, or even ten pounds could be involved. Use a chair or a bench for this workout. Your back should be flat, and one hand should be placed on the bench or chair seat. Maintain a straight arm at your side while using the other hand to hold the dumbbell. Your elbow should be parallel to the side of your body when you bend and raise your arm. After a little moment, release the hold and extend the arm.

HOME EXERCISES

2. Complete 12 dumbbell curls in 3 sets. With a dumbbell in each hand and your arms straight, take a standing position with your feet shoulder-width apart. With both arms raised in front of you, curl them up by bending them at the elbows. Reposition them after a brief moment of holding still.

3. Make three sets of twelve weight pulls using a resistance stretch band. Trace the length of the elastic band with your foot and hold onto both ends. Bend your arms in the same manner as you did with the dumbbells while keeping them straight.

Forcing

1. Do 10 push-ups in 3 sets. When you are kneeling on the ground, place your palms shoulder-width apart on the surface in front of you. Once you maintain a straight back, bend at the knees and descend your upper body towards the floor. Push yourself back up once your chin is almost touching the floor. Once your strength increases, rise off the floor and perform standard push-ups without contacting your knees.

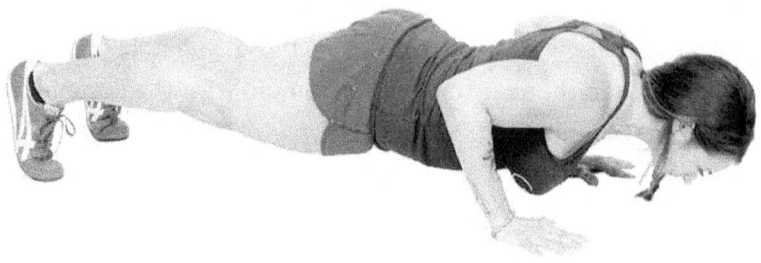

2. Perform three sets of twelve Trice Extensions. Position yourself on your back, arms bent, and hold a pair of dumbbells in each hand. Reaching at nearly full extension with the dumbbells, push them up and away from your body. Return to your chest with them down, and then do so again. Try to maintain as much elbow contact with your body as you can.

3. Complete three sets of twelve shoulder extensions. Taking a standing position, place the dumbbells in your hands and spread your legs wide apart. Lift the weights to your shoulders by bending your arms. Raise them above your head and maintain an almost straight arm position. Returning them to your shoulders should be done slowly.

Exercises for the Abs and Core

A weak core makes it impossible to properly construct your body. Your abs, glutes, and lower back are all part of your core. Your basic strength will be increased by these exercises, which will help you achieve better bodybuilding results.

HOME EXERCISES

Exercises for the Abdominals

1. Perform 10 hip lifts in 3 sets. Assume a floor position where you can look down at your toes with your legs straight up. Keep your arms by your sides and flex your feet as you stand. Elevate your hips several inches off the ground and point your feet upwards without causing any movement or propulsion with your body. When your lower back is on the ground, drop your hips once more.

2. Execute three sets of ten V-Ups. Position yourself on your back, arms at your sides, and legs extended parallel to the ground. Reach for a V-position by raising your head and shoulders simultaneously with your legs. When your legs lift off the ground, so should your arms, lifting them up with them. Go back down to the floor by lowering yourself.

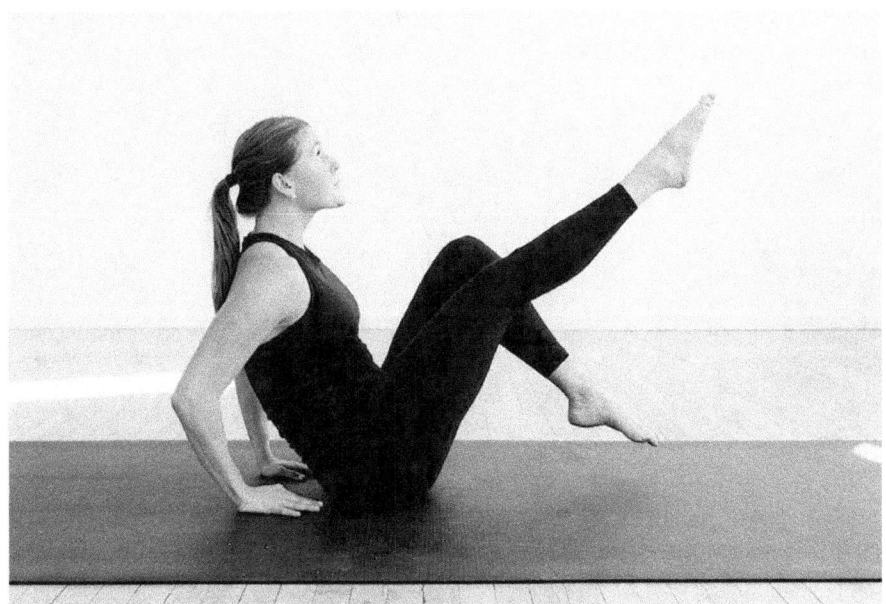

Core Movements

Complete ten repetitions of the downward dog kick in three sets. In an inverted V position, get to all fours and push your hips up and back. Straightening your leg as you lift it, kick your right behind you. After ten reps, rotate to the left leg and perform ten more.

2. For no less than ten seconds, hold a plank three times. Place yourself on your stomach, bending at the elbows, hands flat on the ground, and toes curled beneath your feet. Your back should be flat and your arms should be nearly straight (don't lock your elbows) as you raise yourself into the plank position. Even though it's more challenging for many individuals, you can maintain this position with your elbows on the floor.

Glutei Exercises

1. Perform 16 hip thrusts in three sets. With your knees bent and spaced shoulder-width apart, lie on your back. Maintaining your shoulders on the ground, push your hips toward the ceiling. After three seconds of holding the pose, return to the floor.

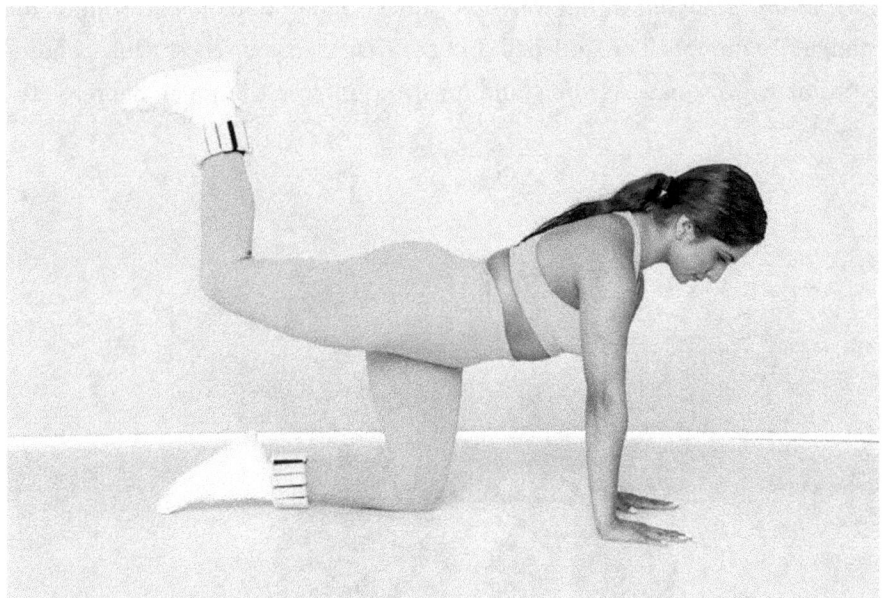

2. Perform ten leg kicks in three sets. Spread your hands shoulder-width apart and get on all fours. Straighten and raise your right leg as far behind you as you can. Without letting the knee touch the floor, bend it and bring it back. Again, kick. Following the right leg, kick the left one.

Lower Body Exercises

The thighs, hamstrings, hips, and quadriceps should all have more strength when you work on your lower body. Muscle growth, balance, and range of motion will all be enhanced by these exercises.

squats

1. Perform 12 squats in three sets. Position your hands on your hips and your legs shoulder-width apart. Drop your body while maintaining a straight back, bending your knees as you progressively drop yourself to the ground. Reach as low as you can go as long as you can push yourself back up to a standing posture.

2. Execute three sets of ten weighted squats. Put both hands in front of you and hold a dumbbell or kettlebell. Lift the weight to your chest while bending your arms to squat. As you stand up straight from the squat, decrease the weight.

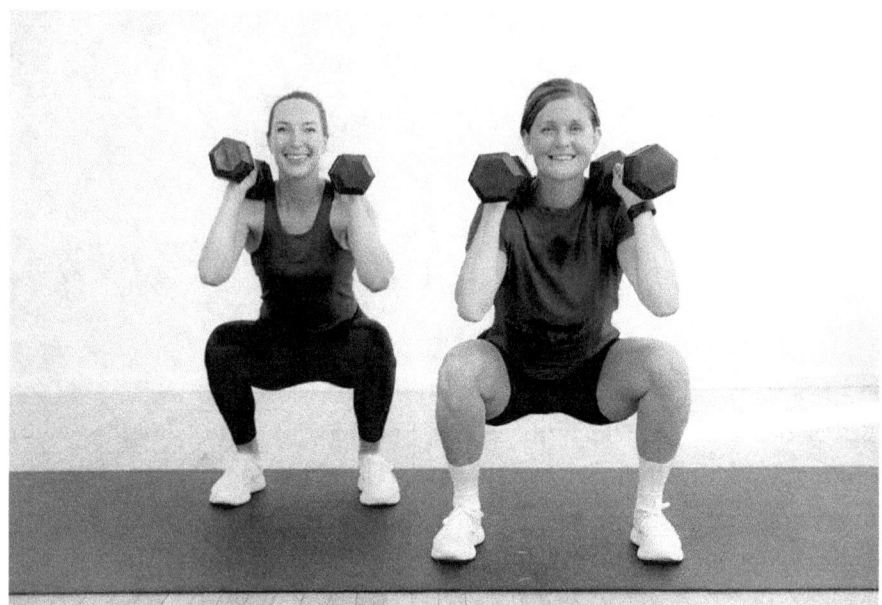

Lurches

1. Perform 10 lunge steps in 3 sets. While keeping your feet together, take a single stride and bend both of your legs until your rear knee almost touches the ground and your leading leg reaches about 90 degrees. Hold your back straight. Legs one by one, alternate between them.

2. Perform ten lunge steps in three sets while carrying a weight. Use both hands to hold one kettlebell or two dumbbells. While the weights in front of you are raised to your chest, finish your lunges.

Jacks That Jump

Most people have performed jumping jacks at some point in their childhood. The glutes, hip flexors, and quadriceps are all nicely worked during this exercise. Along with the shoulders, it targets the stabilizing muscles of the hamstrings, calves, and abdomen.

It's an excellent workout that increases both strength and endurance simultaneously. Proceed and complete three sets of forty jumping jacks. Your daily workout will be well completed with this.

Additional Exercises for the Lower Body

1. Do 10 hip abductions in 3 sets. Support yourself using the back of a chair or a barre while standing with your legs together. Keep your back straight and erect as you swing your right leg out to the side. Replenish it to the earth below. Turn to your left leg after completing ten reps on your right side. You can strengthen and expand your hips with this exercise.

2. Perform ten hip stretches in three sets. Support yourself using the back of a chair or a barre while standing with your legs together. Keep your left leg straight and your back straight as you swing your right leg back behind you. Reposition it so that it is level. Work on your left leg after completing ten reps on your right.

3. Perform 3 sets of 15 toe raises. Grasp the back of a chair or a barre for stability while standing with your legs together. Feel your calves' muscles tense as you raise yourself up onto your toes. Returning to the ground, lower yourself. Reposition yourself onto your toes as soon as possible; don't take a moment to rest.

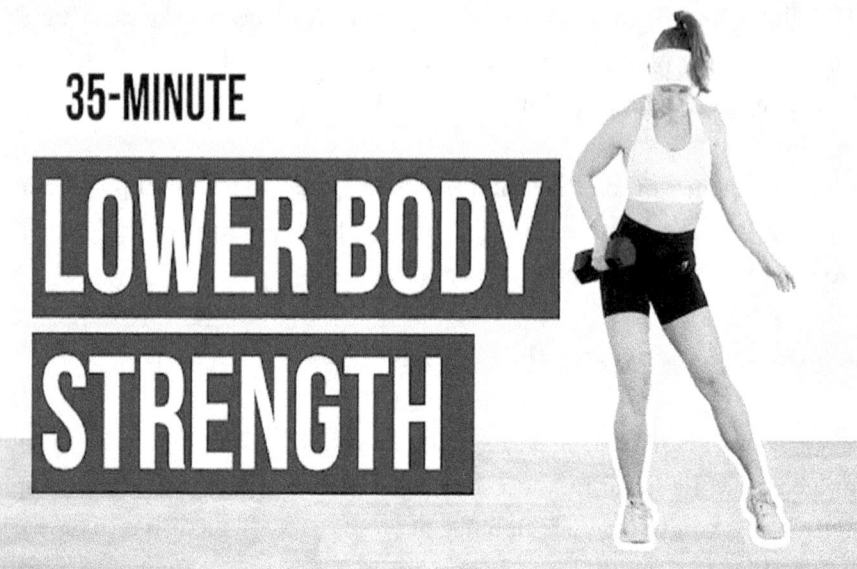

An Example of a 7-Day Schedule

Consider your fitness regimen for entire weeks at a time now that you know what kinds of workouts you may combine with at-home strength training routines. Make careful to include all aspects of strength training in your planning. Furthermore, rest is essential for the healing of your body and muscles. For aspiring bodybuilders, this sample 7-day regimen is a great framework.

First Day – Lower Body

1. First, warm up for ten minutes. Whether you have a treadmill at home or not, take quick walks around your area. You should take an additional five minutes to warm up your legs and hips because today is a lower body workout day. March in three sets and skip in three sets.
2. Execute 12 squats in 3 sets.
3. Perform ten lunge steps in three sets.
4. Complete 3 sets of 10 hip abductions on each leg.

HOME EXERCISES

5. Perform three sets of ten leg-by-leg hip extensions.

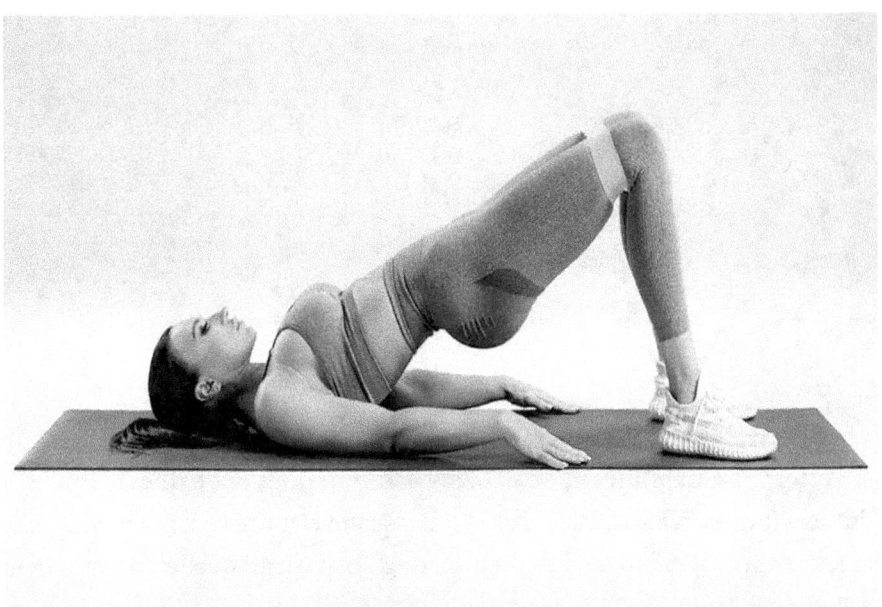

6. Assume the Warrior Pose. In yoga, the legs and lower back are strengthened in this pose. Point the toe of your right foot forward and place it at least three or four feet in front of you. To extend and maintain your balance, turn your left leg as necessary. Enable the front leg to bear the majority of your weight as you raise your arms above your head and gaze at your hands. Switch to place the left leg in front after holding for at least 15 seconds.

Day 2: Upper Body

1. First, warm up for ten minutes. Stride or run. Wrap off your arm workout with three sets of ten arm circles for an additional five minutes.
2. Perform ten pushups in three sets.
3. Work out with a stretch band for three sets of twelve resistance pulls.

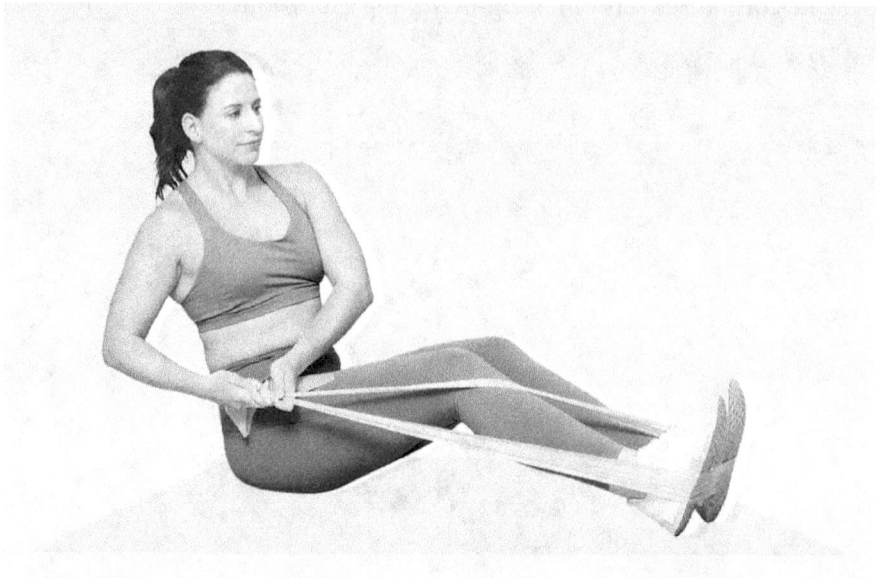

4. Perform 12 arm raises in three sets. Lean your arms out to the sides with a dumbbell in each hand. Raising your arms above your head, make sure they are stretched. Return them to their resting position gradually. Elevate them once more. Hold your arms out straight.

5. Perform three additional sets of ten pushups.

Day 3: Recuperation

Remain mindful of your diet on the day you're taking a break. If at all possible, engage in some unstructured exercise. Jog after your kids at the park, go swimming, or go for a stroll.

Pointing out that muscle growth does not happen during exercise is crucial to maximizing the benefits of bodybuilding exercises. As an alternative, your muscles strengthen and mend during the rest period that follows your workout. Consequently, consuming a balanced diet and getting enough sleep are essential for bodybuilding.

Day 4: Foundation

1. Perform jumping jacks or rope jumping for ten minutes to warm up. Another option is to walk quickly or run in place. For an additional five minutes, perform full circular neck rolls, starting with a nod of affirmation.
2. Execute ten shoulder shrugs in three sets. Elevate your shoulders toward your ears while maintaining a straight stance. Drop them gradually.
3. For at least ten seconds, hold a board in place.
4. Complete 3 sets of 10 pushups.
5. For at least ten seconds, hold another plank.
6. Execute 15 Side Bends in 3 sets. Maintain a shoulder-width distance between your feet. Raising your opposing arm above your head, bend to one side. Return to center, raise other arm over head, and bend the opposite direction.

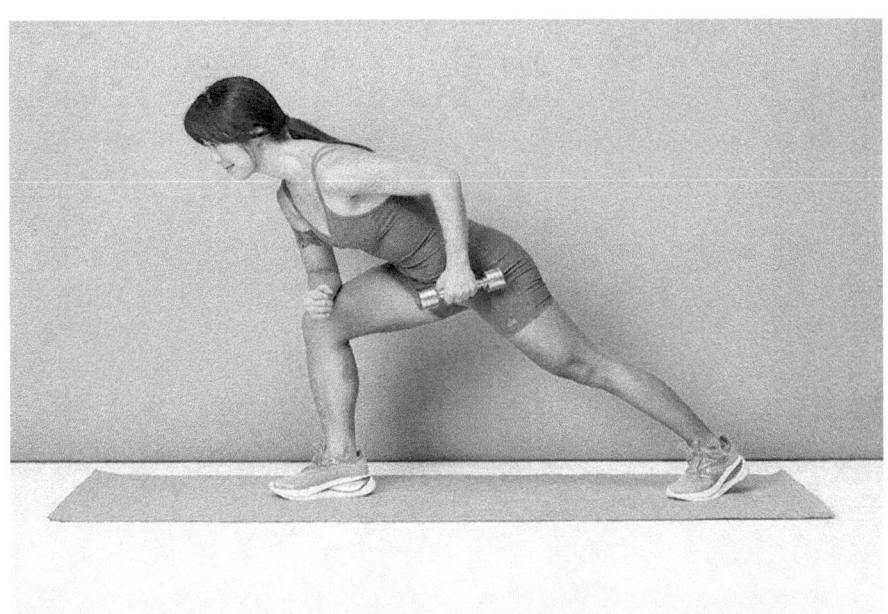

7. For at least ten seconds, hold another plank.

Day 5: Lower Bodies

1. Walk or jog vigorously for ten minutes to warm up. March and skip for an additional five minutes.
2. Perform three sets of twelve chair squats. Although you'll be standing in front of a chair, this exercise is identical to a standard squat. After pushing yourself back up, lower yourself until you are almost in the chair.
3. Perform 3 sets of 15 toe raises.
4. Perform 12 side leg lifts in three sets. Assume a prone position on the ground. With your elbows supporting your upper body, extend your legs. As you raise and lower your left leg to its maximum height, maintain your right leg on the floor. Go to the other side and repeat the process.
5. Perform ten side lunges in three sets. Place your hands on your hips while keeping your feet together. Leap as far to the right as you can without falling and take a substantial step. Returning to the central position requires some pushing. To the left, switch directions.

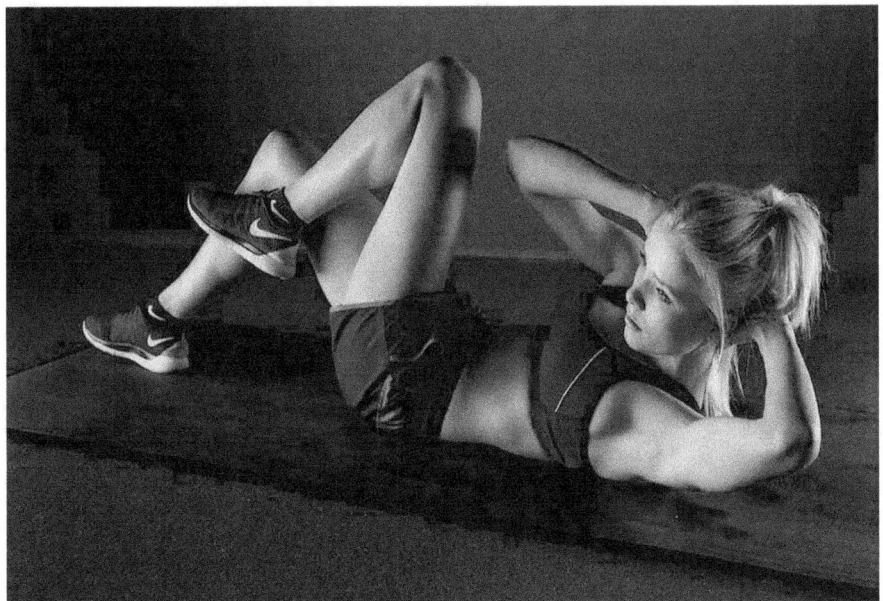

Day 6: Recuperation

After working out your lower body for a second time, you might be experiencing soreness. In order to stretch out your healing muscles, give your body time to rest and go for a leisurely stroll.

Day 7: Lower and Upper Extremities

1. Take ten minutes to jog or walk as a warm-up. Tie your shoes, roll your neck, and roll your shoulders for five minutes.
2. For at least ten seconds, hold a plank.
3. Perform three sets of ten push-ups.
4. Complete 15 hip thrusts in three sets.
5. Perform ten hip lifts in three sets.
6. Complete three sets of ten push-ups.

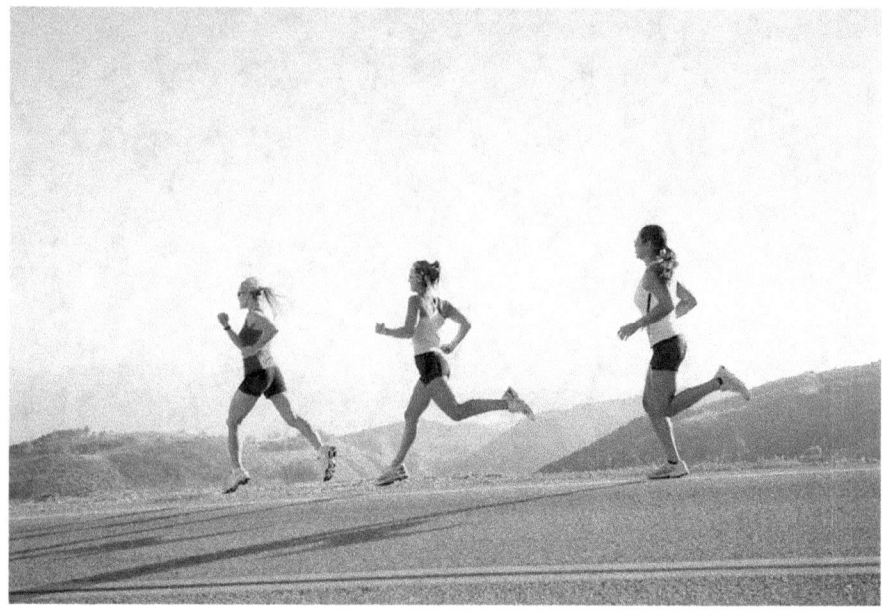

Home Exercises for Strength Training: Variety

Remaining interested is crucial. Repetitions become simpler and you can lift heavier weights (such as dumbbells, kettlebells, or other weights) as your strength and endurance increase. To add to your strength training regimen, you should constantly be searching for new exercises. Designed to be easy enough for beginners, the exercises in this book will help you begin to grasp the physical aspects of your body and your potential for personal development. Try experimenting with other workouts and learning about alternative methods to strengthen and tone your body if you start to get bored or the routines become tedious. Though strength training should be your primary focus, don't forget that modest aerobic exercise has a purpose as well. Your heart, legs, and general physical conditioning will all benefit from it.

You may train your strength at home with these workouts. Joining a gym will help you in your endeavors when you're ready to move on to weight lifting machines. To lay a solid foundation for your training regimen, familiarize yourself with these easy workouts for the time being. For some, working out

HOME EXERCISES

with a friend increases their level of success. In order to ensure that you're on track given your existing talents and growth ambitions, review the strategy and the program if you decide to proceed.

3

Foods to Consume

Foods to Consume When Building Muscle

How strength training and exercise contribute to muscle growth is a key subject in bodybuilding. Your muscle fibers mildly tear and sustain injury when you perform strength or weight training. In the body, satellite cells are a unique sort of cell found close to muscle cells. This activates the satellite cells. The injured muscle fibers are repaired and strengthened by the proliferation of activated satellite cells, which merge with them. Muscle cells are also stimulated by satellite cells to produce new proteins. All of these things work together to strengthen and thicken the regenerated muscles in comparison to their pre-workout state.

It's crucial to consider your diet before starting a strength training program. The nutrients your body needs to develop, repair, and maintain muscle are found in the food you eat. It is more crucial to eat enough to support your peak physical performance than to adhere to a rigid diet and restrict your food and calorie intake. Protein is the key component of a bodybuilding diet since it keeps your metabolism running high and helps you create muscle. This will help you get stronger.

Put Protein First

FOODS TO CONSUME

Your bodybuilding diet's main component will be protein. Food for your cells is protein. Your tissues, especially your muscular tissue, can proliferate and remain healthy thanks to it. The production of hormones and the defense of your blood, skin, and bones are two further functions of protein. Numerous physiological processes slow down and become worse if your diet is deficient in protein. You end up with less muscle, drab skin and hair, and potentially more brittle bones. Protein consumption must be increased while starting a strength training program because you are not only maintaining but also developing a strong and healthy physique.

Foods themselves are the best source of protein. Fish and lean meats like turkey, chicken, cattle, and pork are all OK. Additionally, as well as legumes like beans and tofu, nuts and seeds provide protein. Protein bars, powders, and shakes are added to diets by some people. Incorporating these beneficial protein elements into your diet and giving yourself a burst of energy is a wonderful idea. Nonetheless, in order to prevent hunger, you want to make an effort to consume as much genuine protein as possible. A hearty, high-protein breakfast will provide you with a solid foundation from which to develop, as well as the energy you need to get through your workouts and the rest of the day. Start your day with an egg plate.

There are more benefits associated with using protein in your bodybuilding diet. You won't feel the need to nibble on unhealthy foods during the day since you'll feel fuller. Your metabolism will be positively impacted by the protein, which will also help you burn fat more efficiently. More energy will be available to you as your body transforms the protein into glucose. It has also been demonstrated that diets with a greater protein content and a lower carbohydrate content can help with heart health and weight loss.

There's fat associated with many protein sources. Take that with little concern. Even more so while you're gaining muscle, your body requires the fat. Your body will benefit as long as you consume foods high in healthy fats, like nuts, fish, and oils.

Dietary Practices Before and After Exercise

Your performance will be significantly impacted by what you consume both before and after strength training exercises. If you want to grow muscle and lift weights, have some high-quality carbohydrates and protein before working out. A slice of high-fiber bread topped with scrambled eggs or whole-grain oats topped with fruit and nuts are great options if you enjoy working out in the morning. Pasta or brown rice works well to consume around an hour before beginning strength training if you work out in the afternoon or evening.

Your muscles will recuperate better if you consume some protein after working out. Snack on some fish or some grilled poultry. To nourish and rebuild your muscles in case you're not feeling hungry, consider consuming a protein drink or a protein bar. Be sure to drink plenty of water and steer clear of anything high in glycemic index foods. During your strength training session, this will deplete your energy and make you feel exhausted. Junk food and sugars are sources of empty carbs, which should never be consumed, especially right before or right after exercise.

Holistic Eating

High-protein, high-carbohydrate diets are the norm for bodybuilders who are successful. You won't get any faster or lose weight eating processed foods that are heavy in added fats, sugar, and salt. Make sure you are growing healthy, lean muscle rather than fat if you are going to gain weight during bodybuilding. Making a diet that is wholesome, well-balanced, and appropriate for a strength training program is how to do that.

It's best to eat cleanly. Select proteins, omega-3 fatty acids, and sustainably farmed meats and seafood for your body's construction. Combine lean meat, chicken, turkey, eggs, and fish for your meals. Use full grain bread, pasta, brown rice, and sweet potatoes as essential carbs to complement that protein.

FOODS TO CONSUME

For added fiber and to keep your body in good condition, include some seasonal fruits and leafy green veggies. Go for healthy pro-biotic meals like yogurt and almonds and seeds as your snacking options. By assisting with all of the muscular growth you're attempting to achieve, clean eating can boost your bodybuilding nutrition. When it comes to work, your body will be well-fed. Twenty tasty and nutritious clean eating recipes are included in Chapter 4.

Look out for fad diets. You should avoid drastically reducing your caloric intake, even though losing weight may be one of your fitness goals. Your body cannot grow more muscular and strong if you do that. Pay attention to the kinds of food you're choosing rather than keeping track of calories. More important than the amount of calories or fat grams in your food is what you eat.

Though exercises take precedence, bodybuilding diet is crucial. Lifting weights on a regular and difficult basis is the best way to develop muscle. It will require commitment on your part to work out more frequently and spend time lifting weights. The results you get when you mix that with the appropriate diet will astound you.

4

Healthy Recipes

Healthy Recipes for Eating

In most diets, the focus is on a specific food type, calorie count, or the proportion of fat to protein consumed. It is far easier to eat clean. Eating as naturally as possible can be the epitome of "clean eating." Attempting to consume foods in their natural state is the underlying principle. Choosing raw or unrefined foods is what this entails. Except in cases when you specifically desire them, you are not specifically excluding or including any foods. Nutrient counts, protein requirements, or avoiding veggies that are considered nightshades are unimportant concerns.

Eggs verde for breakfast
  Makes two servings.
  Ingredients:

  1. 4 eggs
  2. two cups little spinach leaves
  3. ½ cup diced green bell pepper; ½ stalk celery; ½ diced zucchini
  4. one tablespoon of almond milk
  5. a single tablespoon of olive oil
  6. According to taste, add salt and pepper.

Guidelines:

1. In a skillet over medium heat, heat the oil. Cook the zucchini, celery, and green pepper for three minutes after adding them.
2. After adding, boil the spinach until it starts to wilt.
3. Add almond milk to the eggs and beat with a fork or whisk. Transfer all the vegetables into the skillet and stir to combine them.
4. Add a dash of spicy seasoning.

Per Serving Nutritional Information

There are 229 calories.
Fat: 17.8 g; Sat Fat: 5.4 g.
6.3 grams of carbohydrate
Fiber: 1.9 g
3 g of sugar
13.1% protein

4 portions of the breakfast casserole Ingredients:

1. Peel and dice four red potatoes.
2. Peeled and chopped one cup of eggplant and one cup of diced butternut squash
3. Garlic cloves four
4. ½ red onion, sliced; 1 chopped red bell pepper; 1 chopped green bell pepper;
5. two cups of broccoli
6. 4 tsp olive oil
7. Fresh rosemary sprig, one
8. Four young basil leaves
9. According to taste, add salt and pepper.

Directions:

1. Set the oven temperature to 375 degrees Fahrenheit. Stir everything until it's well blended, then mix in the olive oil.
2. Bake the vegetables in the oven for forty minutes, or until they are tender and charred.

Information about Nutrition (Per Serving)
Calories : 328
Fat : 14.6 g
Sat Fat : 2.1 g
Carbohydrates : 47.5 g
Fiber : 7.6 g
Sugar : 6.9 g
Protein : 6.7 g

Make Granola on Your Own
Six servings are produced.
Ingredients:

1. A single cup of almonds
2. 1 cup cashews
3. One-half cup of walnuts
4. One-fourth cup of raisins
5. A single cup of oats
6. half a cup of coconut shreds
7. A quarter cup of sunflower seeds
8. A quarter cup of pine nuts
9. Three cinnamon tsp
10. Two cups almond milk

Instructions

1. In order to make sure everything is incorporated, mix all of the dry ingredients together.
2. Divide among 4 bowls, then top each with ½ cup almond milk.

Nutritional Information (Per Serving)
Calories : 471
Fat : 33.5 g
Sat Fat : 5.5 g
Carbohydrates : 36.4 g
Fiber : 6.8 g
Sugar : 11.9 g
Protein : 13.3 g
Sodium : 55 mg

Smoothie with Berries Blast

Ingredients: 1 serving; yield:
One-half cup blueberries
Quarter of a cup strawberries
Half a cup raspberries
A quarter cup of blackberries
One banana, half
one cup of almond milk
1/2 cup of ice

Directions:

1. Everything should be combined in your blender, then mix for 30 seconds on high.

Nutritional Information (Per Serving)

Calories: 240
Fat: 3.9 g
Sat Fat: 0.1 g

Carbohydrates: 51.8 g
Fiber: 12.5 g
Sugar: 30.2 g
Protein: 4.4 g
Sodium: 147 mg

(8) Servings of Carrot Bread Ingredients:

1. Two cups of almond flour.
2. One tsp baking powder
3. A single spoonful of cumin seeds
4. Season with salt to taste.
5. Three huge eggs.
6. Two tsp olive oil
7. A single tablespoon of vinegar made from apple cider
8. Trimmed and grated carrots, three cups
9. 1 tsp freshly peeled and coarsely grated fresh ginger
10. One-half cup of raisins

Directions:

- Oven temperature should be set at 350 degrees Fahrenheit.
- Spread parchment paper inside a loaf pan.
- Combine salt, baking powder, cumin seeds, and almond flour in a big bowl and stir thoroughly.
- Combine the vinegar, olive oil, and eggs in a another bowl and beat thoroughly.
- Mix thoroughly after adding the egg mixture to the flour mixture.
- Fold in the raisins, carrots, and ginger gently.
- Fill the prepared loaf pan with the mixture.
- Cook for approximately one hour, or until a toothpick inserted in the center comes out clean.

Nutritional Information (Per Serving)
Calories: 133
Fat: 8.9 g
Sat Fat: 1.3 g
Carbohydrates: 10 g
Fiber: 2 g
Sugar: 4.9 g
Protein: 4.5 g

One serving of the Southwest Chicken Wrap for lunch
Ingredients:

1. One tortilla made entirely with wheat
2. 6 ounces cooked chicken with diced and shredded carrots, measuring ¼ cup
3. 1/4 cup minced red bell pepper and 1/4 cup cooked black beans
4. Avocado two slices
5. One tsp dry cilantro
6. A tsp of red pepper flakes
7. A quarter of a lime's juice

Directions:

1. Arrange the chicken pieces on the tortilla. Next, add the avocado, beans, pepper, and carrots on top.
2. Add some red pepper flakes and cilantro, and then squeeze some lime over everything. Organize into a wrap.

Nutritional Information (Per Serving)
Calories: 565
Fat: 15.9 g
Sat Fat: 3.4 g
Carbohydrates: 47.2 g

Fiber: 13.6 g
Sugar: 5.6 g
Protein: 60 g
Sodium: 260 mg

One serving of the chicken and rice bowl Ingredients:

1/2 cup of cooked brown rice
1/4 cup of cooked chicken and 1/4 cup of chopped tomatoes
One-half cup of cooked corn
Half a cup of cooked black beans
Just one lime
According to taste, add salt and pepper.

Directions:

1. Top the brown rice with the chicken, corn, and black beans, and mix everything together.
2. Sprinkle the salt, pepper, and fresh tomatoes on top. Add lime juice on top.

Nutritional Information (Per Serving)

Calories: 299
Fat: 3.5 g
Sat Fat: 0.8 g
Carbohydrates: 42.3 g
Fiber: 7.7 g
Sugar: 3.6 g
Protein: 27.7 g

Serves: 2 of the tuna salad.

Ingredients:

1. Four servings of lettuce

2. one tuna can in water
3. one tsp olive oil
4. One teaspoon of newly squeezed lemon juice
5. one-half cup chopped sun-dried tomatoes; one-half cup sliced bell pepper; one-half cup kalamata olives;
6. one sliced celery stalk
7. One-tspn dried oregano

Guidelines:

1. Clean and pat the lettuce dry, then arrange it like a bed on a dish.
2. The tuna, lemon juice, and oregano should be combined in a bowl. When everything is combined, add the veggies.
3. Spoon the tuna mixture onto the lettuce bed after seasoning with salt and pepper.
4. If desired, drizzle on some additional olive oil.

Nutritional Information (Per Serving)
Calories: 232
Fat: 9.3 g
Sat Fat: 1.6 g
Carbohydrates: 16 g
Fiber: 4.3 g
Sugar: 7.9 g
Protein: 23.5 g
Sodium: 633 mg

Sweet Potatoes with Garlic
Ingredients: 1 serving; yield:
Peeled and sliced into thin, round pieces, one medium sweet potato
one tsp olive oil
According to taste, add salt and pepper.
One smashed garlic clove

One teaspoon, minced finely, parsley
1/4 cup grated orange zest

Steps to follow:

1. Set oven temperature to 400 degrees F.
2. Place sweet potato, oil, salt, and pepper in a bowl and combine.
3. Spread the potato slices on a sizable baking pan and drizzle with cooking spray. After baking the potato slice for 10 minutes, flip it over and continue baking for an additional 10 minutes, until it turns golden brown.
4. The potato slices should be taken out and placed in a bowl.
5. Incorporate the chopped parsley, lemon rind, and crushed garlic into a bowl and scatter it over the sweet potato parts. Hot servings are recommended.

Nutritional Information (Per Serving)
Calories: 149
Fat: 4.9 g
Sat Fat: 0.7 g
Carbohydrates: 25.2 g
Fiber: 4.1 g
Sugar: 7.4 g
Protein: 2.6 g

Makes six servings of Turkey and Bean Chili.
Ingredients:

1. Two pounds of ground turkey breast, three cloves of garlic, one minced red onion, one diced green bell pepper, and two tablespoons of olive oil.
2. Half a pound of tomato paste and six fresh tomatoes, seeded and chopped
3. Rinse one cup of red kidney beans, one cup of black beans, one cup of garbanzo beans, and four tablespoons of ground cumin.

4. One teaspoon of coriander powder
5. Chili powder, two tablespoons
6. 1 cup of water
7. ½ cup of salt

Directions:

1. In a large soup pot, simmer the turkey over medium heat for about 10 minutes, or until it is golden. Add chili powder, coriander, and cumin.
2. After taking the turkey out of the pot, add some olive oil. Melt the bell pepper, onion, and garlic.
3. Stir in the salt and the tomatoes. For around ten minutes, let the tomatoes simmer.
4. Reintroduce the meat to the pot after adding the beans and tomato paste.
5. Combine all ingredients by stirring them thoroughly. Use water to cover. Simmer for half an hour with a lid on.

Nutritional Information (Per Serving)

Calories: 745
Fat: 20.4 g
Sat Fat: 4.4 g
Carbohydrates: 76.2 g
Fiber: 20 g
Sugar: 13.7 g
Protein: 67.6 g
Sodium: 758 mg

Eatables

1. Uncooked Egg Whites
2. Makes 12 servings.
3. Six hardboiled and peeled eggs; one cup rinsed capers; one-half cup chopped olives; and one-quarter cup sliced red bell pepper are the

ingredients.
4. a single tablespoon of olive oil
5. According to taste, add salt and pepper.

Directions:

1. Split the eggs lengthwise in half, and then throw away the yolk.
2. Add a pinch of salt and pepper to the beaten eggs.
3. Add the red pepper, olive oil, and olives to a small bowl and use a fork to crush the capers. Blend thoroughly. Put the scoop into the egg whites' holes.

Nutritional Information (Per Serving)
Calories: 49
Fat: 4 g
Sat Fat: 0.9 g
Carbohydrates: 0.9 g
Fiber: 0.3 g
Sugar: 0.3 g
Protein: 2.9 g

Kababs antipasto
Produces 4 servings.
Ingredients:

1. Two celery stalks, cut into big pieces
2. A single cup of white button mushrooms
3. One cup of cubed, cold poultry
4. One cup of heart of artichoke
5. 1 cup of olives
6. pieces of one red pepper
7. pieces of one green pepper
8. 1/2 cup olive oil and 2 cups of cauliflower florets

9. A single spoonful of oregano
10. Taste-tested and add salt and pepper as needed.

In a bowl
1. Combine all the ingredients, stir, and drizzle with olive oil.
2. Take a half-hour break.
3. Arrange the food in a stack above skewers.

Nutritional Information (Per Serving)
Calories: 244
Fat: 17.6 g
Sat Fat: 2.6 g
Carbohydrates: 11.4 g
Fiber: 4.3 g
Sugar: 4.1 g
Protein: 13.2 g

Walnuts and Roasted Seeds
Produces 15 servings.
Ingredients:

1. A single cup of almonds
2. A one cup of walnuts
3. Half a cup almonds
4. A single cup of peanuts
5. OZ of pumpkin seeds and OZ of sunflower seeds
6. A quarter cup of pine nuts
7. One fresh rosemary sprig and two
8. Six young sage leaves
9. A single tsp of cayenne
10. a single tablespoon of olive oil
11. Taste-tested and add salt and pepper as needed.

Directions:

1. Set an oven temperature of 400 degrees Fahrenheit.
2. Using a baking sheet, distribute the nuts and seeds evenly. Add the olive oil, salt, pepper, and cayenne pepper over top. Throw in the sage and rosemary.
3. Roast for approximately twenty minutes in the oven. After removing, let it cool.

Nutritional Information (Per Serving)
Calories: 228
Fat: 20.9 g
Sat Fat: 2.1 g
Carbohydrates: 6 g
Fiber: 3.1 g
Sugar: 1.1 g
Protein: 8.2 g

4 portions of the cinnamon fruit salad
Ingredients:
1 cup blueberries and 2 sliced bananas
Selected one cup of strawberries and one cup of red grapes
1 cup of green grapes
One apple, cored, peeled, and diced; two cups cubed watermelon.
two tablespoons of newly squeezed lemon juice
A single spoonful of cinnamon

Directions:

1. Put all the fruits in a big basin and stir them together. Over all the fruits, squeeze the lemon juice and stir once more.
2. To ensure the flavors meld, let the fruits chill for a minimum of half an

hour.
3. Evenly distribute the cinnamon and savor.

Nutritional Information (Per Serving)

Calories: 186
Fat: 0.8 g
Sat Fat: 0.2 g
Carbohydrates: 47.5 g
Fiber: 6.2 g
Sugar: 33.1 g
Protein: 2.3 g
Sodium: 6 mg

Wonderful Green Juice

Ingredients: 1 serving; yield:
Quarter of an avocado
half a cucumber
1 cup of spinach
Half a cup of fresh mint leaves and one celery stalk
1 tsp finely grated ginger, just off the vine
1 cup of water
1/2 cup of ice

Directions:

1. Toss everything together in a blender until the ice is broken up and the vegetables are well-combined.

Per Serving Nutritional Information

Calories: 242
Fat: 20.1 g
Sat Fat: 4.3 g

Carbohydrates: 16.2 g
Fiber: 9.8 g
Sugar: 2.2 g
Protein: 4.3 g
Sodium: 52 mg

Savory and tart salmon for dinner

Produces 4 servings.

Ingredients:

1. Two tablespoons of chopped scallions and one-half teaspoon of minced fresh ginger root
2. One-third cup finely chopped garlic
3. two tsp olive oil
4. Two tsp balsamic vinegar
5. A single tablespoon of honey
6. quarter of a teaspoon crushed red pepper flakes
7. Season with salt to taste.
8. Salmon fillets, four (6 oz.)

Directions:

1. In a sizable bowl, combine all ingredients, excluding the salmon fillets.
2. Place the salmon on top and liberally brush with marinade. While occasionally tossing, cover and chill to marinate for approximately eight hours.
3. Set a medium-high temperature for the grill.
4. Coat the grill grates in grease. About five inches away from the heat source, place the salmon fillets on the grill grate.
5. Cook for 5 to 10 minutes, turning the salmon fillets once around the halfway point or until they are cooked to your liking.

Nutritional Information (Per Serving)

Calories: 308
Fat: 17.6 g
Sat Fat: 2.5 g
Carbohydrates: 5.5 g
Fiber: 0.2 g
Sugar: 4.5 g
Protein: 33.2 g

Shrimp with Lime-CILANTRO

1. Produces 4 servings.
2. Ingredients:
3. Peeled and deveined, one pound of small to medium shrimp
4. Two tomatoes, cut and seeded.
5. Two limes.
6. Quarter of a cup of raw cilantro
7. half a cup of olive oil
8. According to taste, add salt and pepper.

Directions:

1. Turn the oven's temperature up to 375°F. Mix the tomatoes and shrimp together in a bowl and drizzle with olive oil.
2. Transfer to an ovenproof dish and drizzle with lime juice. Salt, pepper, and cilantro should be added.
3. Cook until shrimp are pink, 20 minutes.

Nutritional Information (Per Serving)

Calories: 242
Fat: 14 g
Sat Fat: 2.2 g

Carbohydrates: 6 g
Fiber: 1.7 g
Sugar: 2.2 g
Protein: 24.5 g

Makes 4 serves of ginger steak.
Ingredients:
8 smashed garlic cloves
Two tsp freshly cut, thin-sliced ginger
A single tablespoon of honey
half a cup of olive oil
According to taste, add salt and pepper.
A 1-and-a-half-pound cut flank steak

Steps to follow:

1. Combine all ingredients, excluding steak, in a big sealable bag.
2. Place the steak in there and liberally brush with marinade.
3. Close the bag and let it marinade in the fridge for approximately a full day.
4. Take the steak out of the refrigerator and allow it to sit at room temperature for approximately fifteen minutes.
5. Turn up the heat to medium-high in a grill pan that has been gently oiled. The steak should be placed in a grill pan after the extra marinade has been disposed of.
6. Continue cooking for 6 to 8 minutes on each side, or until done to your liking.
7. When ready to slice, remove from grill pan and let cool for ten minutes.
8. Slice into appropriate portions using a sharp knife and proceed to serve.

Nutritional Information (Per Serving)
Calories: 471
Fat: 37.9 g

Sat Fat: 1.8 g
Carbohydrates: 7 g
Fiber: 0.3 g
Sugar: 4.4 g
Protein: 24.4 g

Honey-glazed chicken with mustard sauce

Produced in one serving

Ingredients:

1. A quarter-tspn olive oil
2. halves and skins of two boneless chicken breasts
3. A pinch of black pepper and a ¼ teaspoon salt
4. One-fourth cup chicken broth
5. One teaspoon of Dijon mustard
6. a single tsp butter
7. one tsp finely chopped parsley

Steps to follow:

- Preheat the oven to 450°F.
- After adding oil to the chicken, season it with salt and pepper. After putting the chicken in an ovenproof pan, bake it for about ten minutes, or until it has browned.
- After flipping, continue cooking the chicken until the other side is browned. Take out of the pan the chicken.
- Transfer the poultry stock to the pan and allow it to thicken over medium heat. Incorporate the butter, parsley, and mustard.
- Cover the chicken with the mustard sauce and warm it up.

Per Serving Nutritional Information

Calories: 414
Fat: 21.4 g

Sat Fat: 5.4 g
Carbohydrates: 1.2 g
Fiber: 0.6 g
Sugar: 0.3 g
Protein: 52.1 g
Sodium: 1251 mg

Curry with meatballs; yields 6 servings.
Meatball ingredients:

1. one pound of turkey that is lean.
2. two whisked eggs
3. ¼ cup freshly cut basil leaves; ¼ teaspoon finely chopped fresh ginger; three tablespoons minced red onion;
4. chopped finely four garlic cloves
5. Minced and seeded jalapeño pepper
6. One tablespoon of paste for red curry
7. 1 tsp of fish sauce
8. Two teaspoons of coconut oil
9. Season with salt to taste.

To Curry:

1. 4 minced garlic cloves, 1 chopped red onion, 1 minced jalapeño pepper with seeds, and ½ teaspoon of fresh ginger
2. Two tsp red curry paste.
3. One coconut milk can (14 oz.)
4. a pair of teaspoons of fresh lime juice
5. According to taste, add salt and pepper.

Directions:

1. For the meatballs, combine all the ingredients (except the oil) in a large bowl and stir until thoroughly mixed. Form the mixture into tiny balls.
2. Use a big skillet over medium heat to melt coconut oil. Cook for 3 to 5 minutes, or until meatballs are golden brown on all sides, after adding them. Empty the meatballs into a dish.
3. Simmer the onion for three minutes in the same skillet along with a dash of salt.
4. Saute for one minute after adding the jalapeño, garlic, and ginger.
5. Saute the curry paste for one minute.
6. After the meatballs and coconut milk are added, boil gently. Simmer covered for approximately ten minutes on low heat.
7. Add a squeeze of lime juice to the dish.

Nutritional Information (Per Serving)
Calories: 370
Fat: 29.5 g
Sat Fat: 20.8 g
Carbohydrates: 9.8 g
Fiber: 2.2 g
Sugar: 3.7 g
Protein: 19 g

5

Tips for Novices

Tips for Novices in Strength Training

It's only normal to be excited when you decide to start a strength training regimen. Still, it's critical to pace oneself. Avoid going too hard too soon and burning out or risking injury during your early exercises. These are a few beginner's suggestions for strength training that will enable you to dedicate your time and attention to the exercise without having inflated expectations of yourself.

First tip: Take Your Time.

At first, you have only yourself to compete with, even if you eventually make your way onto the competitive circuit. Ease into the process and allow yourself to get better with time is the aim. Seeking to outshine a workout partner who also engages in strength training, or measuring yourself against someone who have been lifting weights for years, are pointless.

Remember to keep your attention on yourself and your goals. Work out as many times as you are comfortable, starting out slowly. You'll likely feel let down, sore, and unable to continue if you promise yourself that you'll lift weights for two hours a day, seven days a week. Make tiny, achievable objectives. Perhaps start out with just two days per week or a small weight loss. Initiate at a reduced tempo and attempt to increase it.

Advice 2: Gradually Up the Intensity

Gradually up the intensity as soon as you discover a comfortable and sustained pace. Once you feel that lifting is getting easier, go from a 10-pound weight to a 15-pound weight and continuing adding more. Utilize your repetitions in the same way. Increase the number of lifts from eight to ten, twelve, and fifteen. You'll discover how to assess your own emotions and the maximum amount of weight that your muscles can support. Avoiding injury and discouragement from trying to increase too much too quickly can be achieved by proceeding cautiously. Relax and have faith in your body. Strength training is a long-term fitness program; it's not a competition. Every two weeks, increase your weight.

Step 3: Pay Attention to Free Weights

You may be mesmerized by intricate machinery and sophisticated devices, depending on the type of gym you attend. You can even use free weights at home, so keep in mind that they're the ideal way to begin a strength training program. As you gain strength and require a more challenging exercise, you can transition to the machines from barbells and dumbbells, which will help you develop a strong base of lean muscle mass. To lift weights wherever you are, get some free weights in different sizes and weight ranges.

Fourth Tip: Take Vacancies

An abundance of novices are so enthusiastic about their ambitions that they wish to work out daily. But your muscles will take those days off to heal and rebuild themselves so that you can train them out again the following week. Your body needs rest. To train your legs one day and your chest and arms the next, isolate the different muscle groups. Three or four days a week should be your goal to stick to. You won't suffer from overuse soreness or injury, but you'll have enough of a schedule to become used to doing out every other day.

Fifth Tip: Acquire Correct Form

Consider working with a personal trainer or teaming up with someone who knows proper form if you're unsure about what or how to lift. You'll find it difficult to overcome negative habits if, as a novice, you pick up bad techniques. For a while, unless you can achieve and sustain the proper form, you might need to continue with lower weight levels. Nevertheless, as you advance, it will be worthwhile.

Tip 6: Put safety first.

A companion who can spot you is ideal for doing out with, especially when doing large lifts. When lifting weights greater than you have previously lifted, put on a safety belt and don't be embarrassed to ask for assistance. Those who are new to bodybuilding can get valuable knowledge from more seasoned competitors, and most bodybuilders are happy to share their knowledge and insights. For hand protection, some bodybuilders use gloves. Be cautious when working out and take all the necessary safety precautions.

Tip 7: Be Mindful of Your Nutrition

Food has a big part in how you lift, as you are well aware. Thus avoid junk food, consume a lot of protein, and drink plenty of water before, during, and after exercise. Avoid caloric restriction and ensure that your intake of food is sufficient to fuel your weightlifting activities.

Tip 8: Look into Compound Motions

At first, make things simple. Make your workouts simple enough. Instead, focus on the fundamentals. Deadlifts, bench presses, shoulder lifts, and squats should all be part of your weekly routine. Before moving on to more advanced lifts that target the specific muscle groups you need to strengthen, concentrate on the fundamentals.

Advice 9: Comply with Your Schedule

Stay with your regimen once you've established one. More than anything else, consistency will yield better outcomes for you. You're getting a decent workout as long as you can train every muscle group once a week and feel like you've pushed yourself without going too far.

10th Tip: Adopt a Comprehensive Perspective

It takes strong general health to perform strength training. Avoid letting alcohol, smoke, or drugs undermine your plans. In addition to learning stress management techniques, make sure you receive adequate sleep each night. More than just weightlifting is required to develop an exceptional physique. A dedication to general well-being is required.

Here are ten novice strength training suggestions that will increase your chances of developing a stronger physique. Investigate what suits you best and then follow them. Both your bodybuilding success rate and results will rise as a consequence.

To sum up

For women, there are many advantages to strength training. Your daily routine and degree of fitness can be catered to. You'll be shocked at how rapidly your range of motion increases when you start with modest weights and a few repetitions. It is my goal that this book will assist you in burning fat and calories and developing a toned, slender physique.

Lastly, I would want to express my gratitude for reading my book. Would you please take a moment to write a review on Amazon and share your thoughts if you liked the book? It would be very valued!

6

Beginning Yoga

The Overview of Yoga

Yoga harmonizes the body, mind, and soul via relaxation. Practitioners are able to reconnect with the environment and themselves through a series of breathing and stretching exercises. Originating in ancient India, yoga disciplines consist of a combination of spiritual, mental, and physical practices. This is a common way to relieve tension and anxiety through exercise, and it belongs to one of the six mainstream schools of Hindu philosophy. Presently, millions of people worldwide engage in and enjoy yoga practice. A wide range of yoga schools exist, as well as practices and approaches deeply ingrained in Buddhism, Jainism, and naturally, Hinduism.

Yoga's foundational ideas

A unique set of objectives, convictions, and tenets guide the life of every yoga practitioner. That being said, there are a few elements that are applicable to all styles and skill levels of yoga. One of the guiding concepts is relaxing. It's not like high impact running, jumping, or lifting like other forms of exercise. Relaxing your body, mind, and spirit will be your main priority. It requires effort to relax your muscles and let go of stress. Your body will become more relaxed and flexible via the training you receive.

Breathing correctly is another principle. As a spiritual and ascetic practice of Hinduism, yoga instructs practitioners in the regulation and control of their breathing. In addition to properly conversing with your ideas and expanding your mind's eye, the latter is crucial for lowering daily stress, worry, and tension.

Yoga is really helpful in weight loss since it incorporates another important concept, which is nutrition. You will become aware of the fuel you are giving your body when you strive to maintain balance in both your life and spirit. Eating fresh, healthful food is meant to nurture both your body and mind. For serious yoga practitioners, a light and strong body is a prerequisite, and eating well will help you reach your goals more quickly. Last but not least, yoga values meditation. In the process of reuniting the body and soul as a single, cohesive entity, this approach clears the mind of conceptual clutter.

An Overview of Yoga's Past

While there is disagreement among practitioners over the exact beginnings of yoga, the majority of them give India credit for around 3000 B.C.. The Indus Valley is the location of stone-carved depictions of individuals doing yoga. Thousands of years before any current, contemporary, or social improvements, these pictures depict the initial yoga poses and techniques. Maintaining balance between the heart and soul can be achieved through yoga, which remains a crucial practice today. Every "yogi" (practitioner, disciple, instructor, or guru) aspires to attain spiritual enlightenment as their path. Fundamentally, this is the recognition of a higher force, which for some people may be God and for others may be the natural world or the stars.

The Yoga Path with Eight Limbs

Patanjali's Yoga Sutra contains information on the eight limbs of yoga. This system of fundamental principles, known as ashtanga, was created to assist practitioners in leading lives that are meaningful and fulfilling.

These limbs teach virtuous ethics, morals, and self-discipline as a route to heavenly illumination. In a similar vein, they assist us in raising our level of longevity and health while addressing the spiritual components of our nature. Following Patanjali, these are the eight limbs of yoga:

Yuki

Yama refers to the first limb of yoga. Our attention is drawn to our actions and the proper way to behave in daily life thanks to this discipline. Likewise, it imparts knowledge on our moral compass and principles of ethics. Known as the Golden Rule, yamas are intended to be universal standards of behavior. Obviously, this means treating people how you would like to be treated. regard for oneself, for instance, stems from regard for others.

In Niyama

Niyama refers to the second limb. Self-control and adherence of spiritual practices are the main foci of this limb. In order to observe spiritual health and well-being, for instance, one must attend a house of worship and say grace before meals. Sitting down to meditate on a daily basis or go for solitary walks can also help you connect with your inner self and discover your purpose for being on this earth.

With Asana

Asanas refers to the third limb. In yoga, which views the body as the temple of the spirit, these are the poses that are practiced. Asanas are believed by yogis to promote spiritual development as well as better daily health, discipline, and attention. It is also through asanas that we can focus and meditate for peace, harmony, and joy on the inside as well as the outside.

Asana Yama

Pranayama refers to the fourth limb. This is basically the practice of breath control, which aims to regulate and master our breathing. Together with learning how healthy breathing may enhance our minds and emotions, we also discover the link between breath and life. The term "pranayama" means "life force extension," and it is a practice that yogis believe nourishes and revitalizes the body, mind, and soul. You have the option to incorporate this technique into your regular yoga practice or work on it alone.

Pratyahara

We call it Pratyahara, the fifth limb of yoga. Retraction from the outer world, its stimulation, and its surroundings is what this basically entails. Pratyahara is an attempt to consciously achieve a kind of separation from our senses as a kind of sensory transcendence. We focus our whole attention inward when we use this method. Because of this, we are able to take a step back from the daily grind and examine ourselves within. Understanding our behaviors and cravings also helps us recognize how detrimental they may be to our general health, wellbeing, and well-being.

Maharashtra

In yoga, dharana is the sixth limb. The idea that every yoga limb or level sets us up for the next is crucial to understand. Considering this, pratyahara comes before dharana, or concentration. This limb will help us overcome the various stimuli, diversion, and meandering ideas that nag at our regular thinking. Proper practices for meditation are also modeled by this type of concentration. We acquire more capacity for focus and learn how to slow down our thought processes through Dharana. This helps us take charge of our thoughts and brains rather than letting them rule us. You'll enter a state of sustained meditation on a daily basis by learning this technique and becoming proficient in it.

Dharam Vir

Consisting of an unbroken stream of focus, dhyana is the seventh limb of yoga. One term for dhyana is meditation, and another for dharana is focus. There's a thin line separating these limbs, but these stages are also entangled. In contrast to dhyana, which is awareness without focus, dharana is the practice of achieving one-pointed attention. When practicing dhyana, you have little to no ideas and your mind is silent.

This point also sees you gain greater strength and endurance. In contrast, yoga emphasizes discipline, daily instruction, and following rather than perfection. It follows that while no endeavor is ever insurmountable, it's acceptable to move on with your life if you are unable to accomplish a goal. Every yoga level, regardless of experience level, offers psychological and physical advantages.

Samadhi

Samadhi is yoga's eighth and last stage, or limb. A practitioner experiences a connection to the Divine in this natural state of ecstasy. Your perspective and attention are now integrated with the self—itself—in what is also regarded as the final stage of meditation. Keep in mind that yoga can only be experienced, not "mastered" in the traditional sense. All phases where spiritual enlightenment could transpire are covered by this.

Different Styles of Yoga

The greatest benefits from yoga can be obtained by selecting a style that is appropriate for your skills and objectives, as there are many different forms of yoga. Beginners can learn yoga effectively using hatha yoga. This gentle method of breathing and stretching is a great option if you're new to yoga or are just starting out. It will be soothing and revitalizing for you.

The advantages of yoga

Your mental, emotional, and physical health will all benefit greatly from yoga practice. Utilizing it will help you feel lighter, stronger, and younger. Stretching your body, burning calories, and improving your appearance are just a few benefits; it also provides you with a comprehensive approach to physical fitness and wellbeing. Yoga teaches your body to be free-flowing, adaptable, and in harmony with your emotions. For individuals who wish to concentrate on breathing, stretching, and reaching the elusive state of inner serenity, it might be an excellent addition to an already established fitness regimen.

Yogic Benefits for Losing Weight: Physical

Few people know how effective yoga may be as a way to burn calories. Not like running, basketball, or cross training, it won't make you leap around and perspire. If you practice yoga for thirty or sixty minutes a day, you will, nevertheless, consistently burn calories. Approximately 300 calories can be burned in an hour by practicing Hatha yoga poses and positions, even if you are just starting out. You can burn even more calories if you hike up the intensity and practice a more vigorous style of yoga, like Vinyasa or Ashtanga. There are calories to be burned from any type of movement.

Another important benefit of yoga for weight loss is having a greater awareness of your body. Paying attention to your body's movements and actions is necessary for every stance and position. You'll be acutely aware of the manner in which the many components of your body function together, as well as feeling every muscle and limb.

A major advantage of yoga is increased flexibility. You'll improve your balance and mobility as a result of all the stretching you undertake. Your breathing and movement will become more effortless, and your posture will also get better. It may not seem like this would be crucial for weight loss, but it is. Your degree of physical fitness automatically rises when you have greater ease of movement. Your body continues to burn fat as a result of this movement. Superior flexibility equates to increased fitness. When you are completing even basic tasks, you will realize that you feel better and look better in your clothes.

Yoga's Advantages for Losing Weight: Thought

In yoga, mental, emotional, and physical fitness are combined. Thinking positively plays a major role in weight loss success. As you practice yoga on a daily basis, you are teaching your mind to use positivity and intention as powerful tools for weight loss. You can use the time to imagine yourself as stronger, leaner, and healthier as you are extending and maintaining positions. Weight loss will come more easily to you if you live in an expectation-filled state. Yoga can assist you in connecting with and utilizing your purpose to lose weight, as the mind is an effective tool in this fight.

More than just avoiding bad food and upping physical activity, weight management also involves managing stress. An emotional imbalance can lead you to unhealthy habits when you feel stressed or overwhelmed. Your body and mind are kept at ease by yoga, which also teaches you how to guide yourself back to a peaceful condition when stress threatens. You'll stay balanced and optimistic with that mindfulness.

One powerful, uplifting method to transform your life is through yoga. The way you look and feel will improve right away, regardless of whether you're starting from scratch or expanding on an existing practice.

7

Yoga Program

Beginner's Two-Week Yoga Program:

Week One

Starting a yoga practice doesn't require any special skills, and it may be done practically anyplace without any equipment. For novices and those who would like to practice at home, these factors make this a great exercise. Wearing yoga pants, leggings, or shorts with a shirt that is cozy but not too baggy is beneficial, even if there aren't many strict rules when it comes to attire for yoga. As well as practicing on a mat or towel, you should also practice barefoot.

Using this two-week yoga training plan for beginners, you will study and practice a new, basic pose every day for two weeks, with Sundays serving as a review of all the subjects covered. The opening and closing poses for every yoga session will be taught to you on the first day of classes.

Easy and Corpse Pose for the First Week's Monday

Called the Easy stance, this is the first stance to master. You will start each session by striking this stance.

YOGA PROGRAM

1. Put your legs out in front of you, crossed at the shins, and start sitting.
2. With both feet beneath the knee of the person opposite you, spread your knees wide and pull your legs in toward you.
3. Place your palms up or down on your knees to rest your hands.
4. Fourth, sit up straight by maintaining an even weight distribution across your hip bones.
5. Stretch your spine and elongate your head and neck.
6. Extend your chest while lowering your shoulders backward.
7. Taking deep breaths, hold this stance for fifteen minutes.

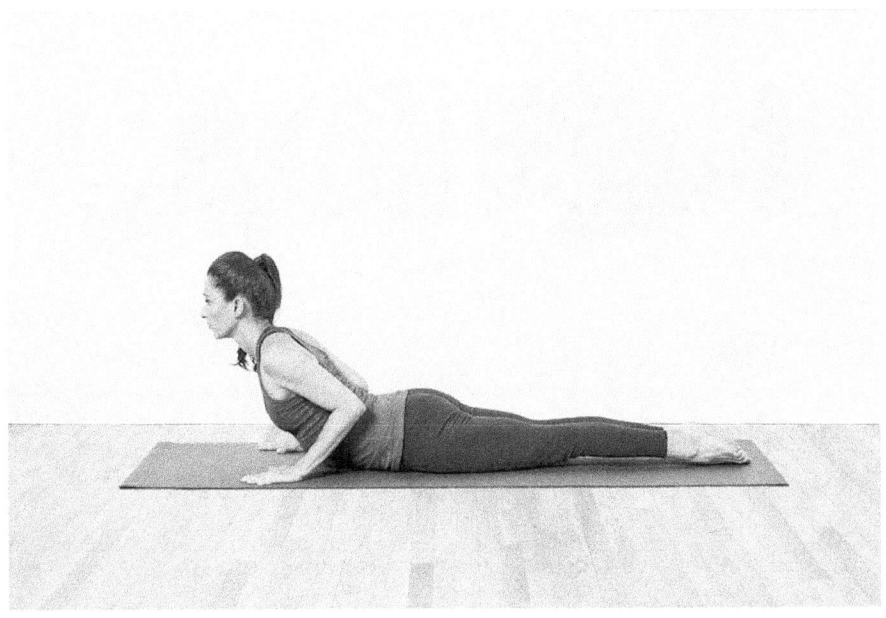

Corpse Pose is the second pose that needs to be learned. This is the posture you will finish each session with because it is thought to be the most crucial to learn.

1. With your arms six inches from your sides and your palms facing up, lie on your back.

2. Breathe organically.
3. Close your eyes and start deliberately letting go of every muscle in your body, starting from your head and ending at the base of your feet).
4. Continue holding this position for a maximum of fifteen minutes.

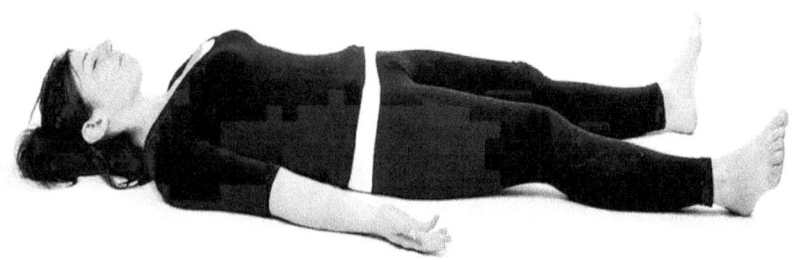

Tuesday: Handstand in mountain position

1. Hold the Easy Pose for five minutes to start.
2. Position yourself tall and place your feet hip-width apart to begin the Mountain Pose.
3. Maintain a comfortable stance, balanced weight, and your arms by your sides.
4. After inhaling deeply, raise your hands and extend your fingers skyward.
5. Breathe easily as you hold for up to a minute.
6. Take a few more variations of the stretch while standing with your hands by your sides.

7. Close by spending five minutes in corpse pose.

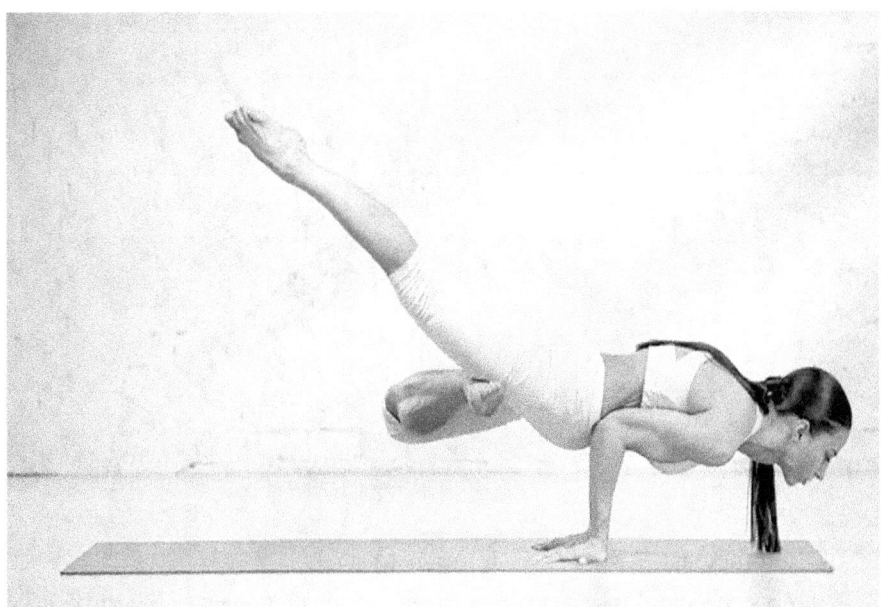

Warrior Pose on Wednesday

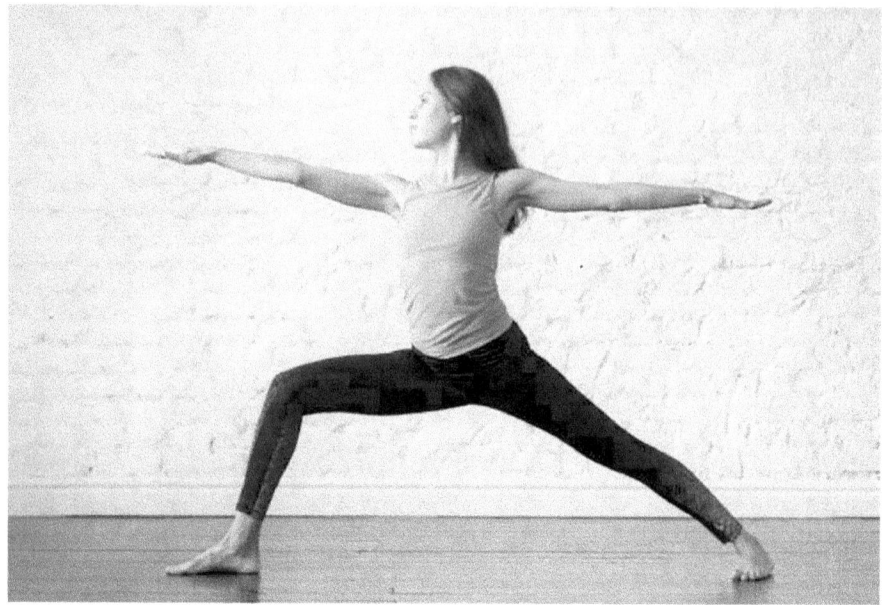

1. Hold the Easy Pose for five minutes to start.
2. Step two: Stand with your feet three to four feet apart to begin Warrior Pose.
3. Slightly turn your left foot inward while rotating your right foot 90 degrees.
4. Extend yourself to your sides, palms down, while maintaining your shoulders down and your hips relaxed.
5. Maintaining the right knee above the ankle, bend it to a 90-degree angle.
6. Take a minute to maintain the stance while gazing out over your right hand.
7. Trade places, then repeat as desired number of times.
8. Complete a five-minute corpse pose.

On Thursday, practice downward dog

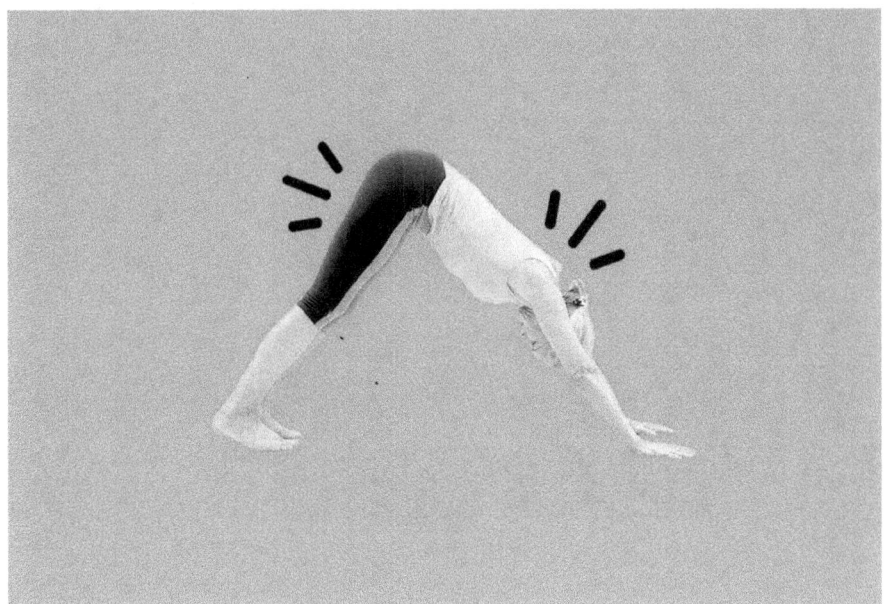

1. Hold the Easy Pose for five minutes to start.
2. Go to the floor on all fours to begin Downward Dog.
3. Assume that your knees are beneath your hips and your hands are beneath your shoulders.
4. With your palms flat on the ground, slowly extend your fingers and walk your hands forward.
5. To create the appearance of an inverted V, raise your hips and curl your toes under while slightly bending your knees.
6. Taking three deep breaths, maintain this stance while breathing easily. As often as you'd want, you can repeat the entire process.
7. Close by spending five minutes in corpse pose.

<u>Friday: Cobra Pose</u>

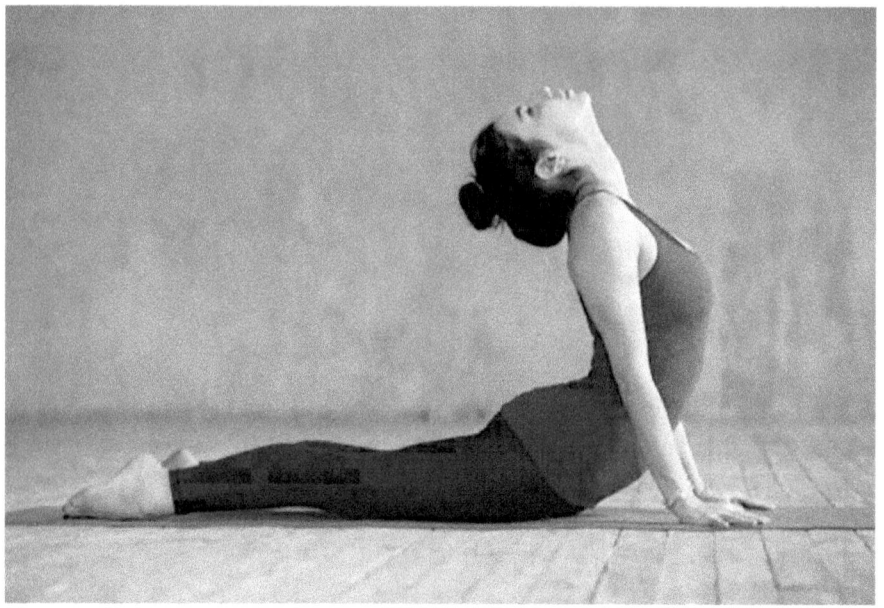

1. Hold the Easy Pose for five minutes to start.
2. Stand tall and straight with your arms by your sides to begin the Tree Pose.
3. Transfer weight to your left leg and tuck your foot inside your left thigh while maintaining a forward hip angle.
4. Stand upright, then raise your hands to your front in the posture of prayer with your palms facing each other.
5. Take a deep breath, extend your arms over your shoulders, and maintain the position for 30 seconds with your palms facing apart.
6. Bend arms, then switch to the other side.
7. Repeat as often as desired, switching between the left and right sides.
8. Complete a five-minute corpse pose.

Saturday: Forward Bend

YOGA PROGRAM

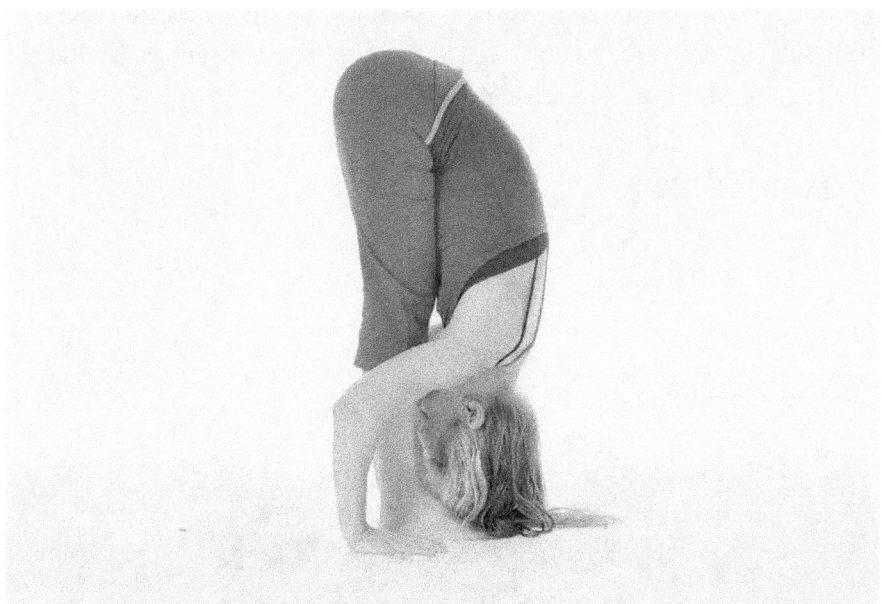

1. Hold the Easy Pose for five minutes to start.
2. To begin Bridge Pose, place your arms at your sides and your hands flat on the ground while resting on your back.
3. Put your knees bent and squarely over your heels while keeping your feet on the ground.
4. Upon exhaling, elevate your hips till your thighs are parallel to the floor by pressing your feet into the ground.
5. Press down with your arms while holding your hands beneath your lower back.
6. Maintain the stance for a minute, then switch it up however many times you'd want.
7. Close by spending five minutes in corpse pose.

Sunday: Examining the First Week and Posing the Child

Easy Pose should be held for one minute at a time. Next, move on to Mountain, Warrior, Downward Dog, Tree, and Bridge poses, holding each for a moment.

As you perform the Warrior and Tree poses, make sure to spend a minute on each side. After the review, proceed to the new pose for Sunday, Child Pose, and finish in Corpse Pose as usual.

The Child's Position

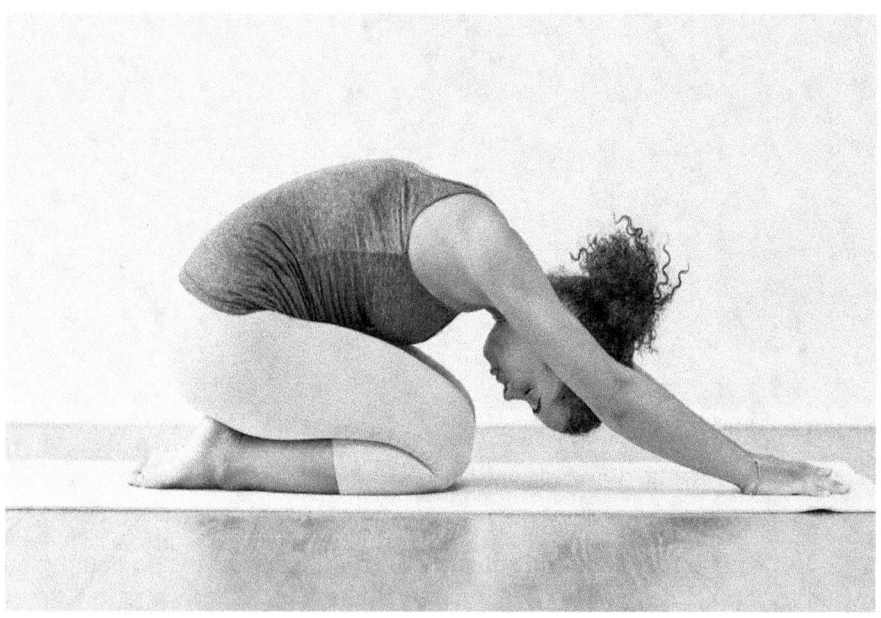

1. After reviewing Week 1, sit up straight on your heels to begin Child's Pose.
2. Exhale and place your forehead on the ground in front of you.
3. While extending your arms straight in front of you, lower your chest to your knees as near to your comfort level as possible.
4. Plant your hands palm down on the earth.
5. Taking deep breaths, hold this stance for one minute, and repeat as many times as you choose.
6. Conclude by spending a minute in corpse pose.

8

Yoga Training Schedule

Beginner's Two-Week Yoga Training Schedule:

Week 2

One new stance will be taught to you every day for the second week, and at the end of the week, you will review every pose you learned.

Triangle Pose on Monday

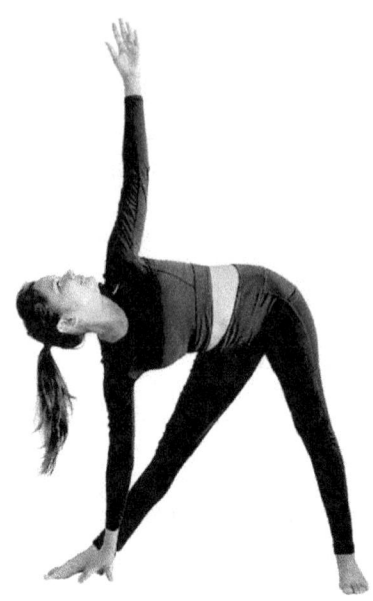

1. Hold the Easy Pose for five minutes to start.
2. Stand upright, place your feet shoulder-width apart, and extend your arms out to your sides to begin Triangle Pose.
3. With your left foot at a 45-degree angle and your right foot out to 90 degrees, turn them both.
4. Maintaining erect legs, touch your right hand to your right foot.
5. Exhale five times while raising your left hand to the sky and looking up past it.
6. Continue the same on the other side.
7. Repeat as often as desired, switching between the left and right sides.
8. Complete a five-minute corpse pose.

Dog facing upward on Tuesday

YOGA TRAINING SCHEDULE

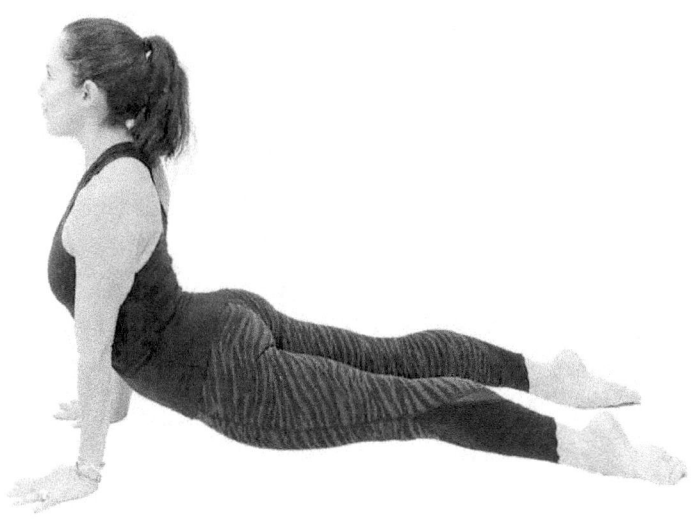

1. Hold the Easy Pose for five minutes to start.
2. Laying face down on the floor, initiate the Upward Facing Dog pose.
3. Immediately beneath your shoulders, lay your hands flat with the palms facing down.
4. Keep the tops of your feet on the ground as you extend your legs behind you.
5. Pinch your buttocks and tighten your pelvic floor by tucking your hips down.
6. Firmly grasp the earth with your hands while keeping your hips on the ground and lifting your chest off the floor.
7. Hold for one minute, then let go and repeat as many as desired.
8. Complete a five-minute corpse pose.

<u>Wednesday: Twist while seated.</u>

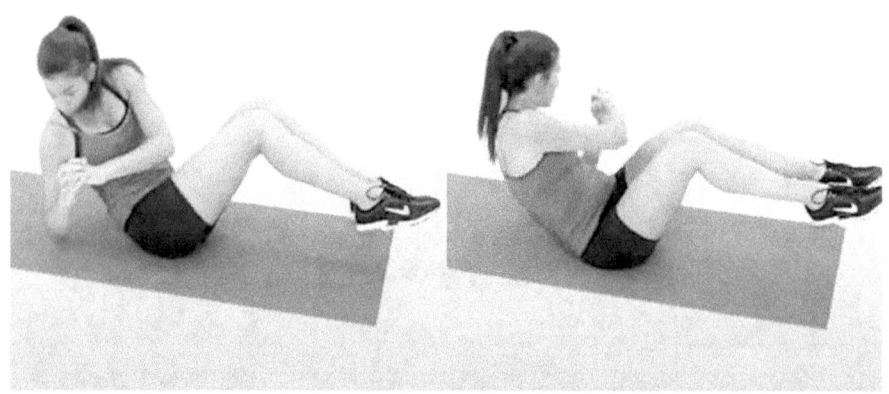

1. Hold the Easy Pose for five minutes to start.
2. Lean forward onto the floor and extend your legs straight in front of you to begin the Seated Twist pose.
3. Cross over and place your right foot outside of your left leg.
4. Bend left knee while extending right knee toward the sky.
5. Slide your left elbow outside of your right knee while maintaining your right hand on the floor for stability.
6. From your abdomen, rotate to the right as far as feels comfortable, keeping both sides of your buttocks on the floor.
7. Hold for a maximum of one minute.
8. Turn to the other side.
9. Repeat as many times as you like, switching between the left and right side.
10. Finally, spend five minutes in corpse pose.

Thursday: Pose like a Pigeon

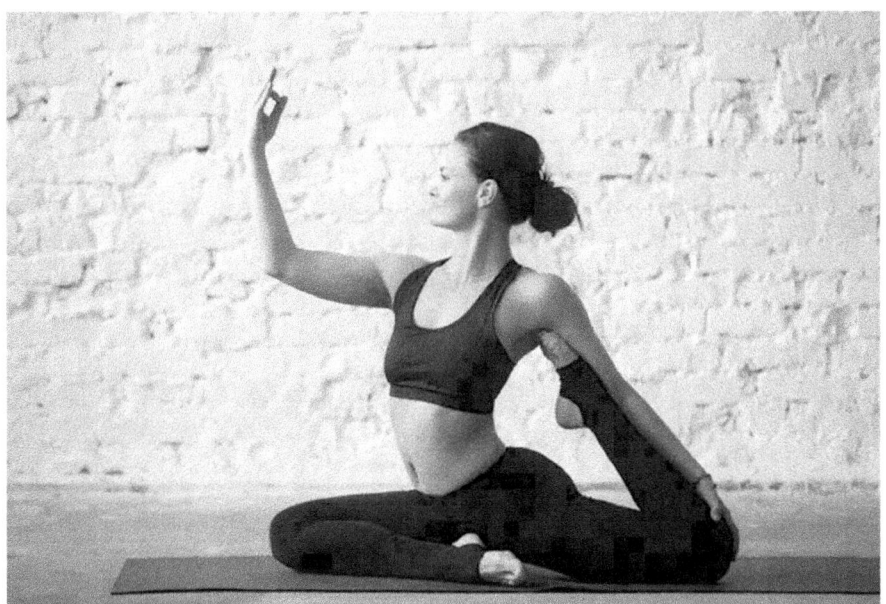

1. Hold the Easy Pose for five minutes to start.
2. Place your palms down, right under your shoulders, to begin Pigeon Pose from a push-up position.
3. Bring the left knee up to the level of your shoulder. In relation to your right hip, your left heel should be.
4. Lift your chest and dig your hands into the ground before reclining.
5. Maintain the stance for a maximum of a minute.
6. Make the appropriate side switch.
7. Repeat as often as desired, switching between the left and right sides.
8. Complete a five-minute corpse pose.

Dolphin Pose on Friday

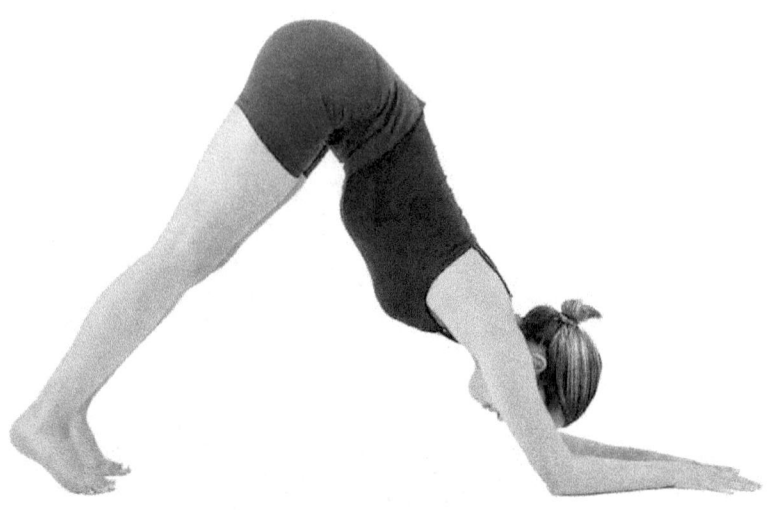

1. Hold the Easy Pose for five minutes to start.
2. Assume Downward Dog Pose to begin Dolphin Pose 2.
3. Lie on your forearms on the ground in the downward dog position.
4. Hold your hands shoulder-width apart while spreading your fingers widely.
5. Breathe deeply and hold the position for a minute while pressing your forehead to the ground.
6. Close by spending five minutes in corpse pose.

Saturday: Pose in half a wheel

1. Hold the Easy Pose for five minutes to start.
2. To begin the Half Wheel Pose, assume Bridge Pose.
3. Elevate your hips to the maximum in the bridge position, then shift your weight off your heels and onto your toes alone.
4. Remain flat-palmed and keep your arms positioned on the ground. For a maximum of one minute, maintain this posture.

5. Close by spending five minutes in corpse pose.

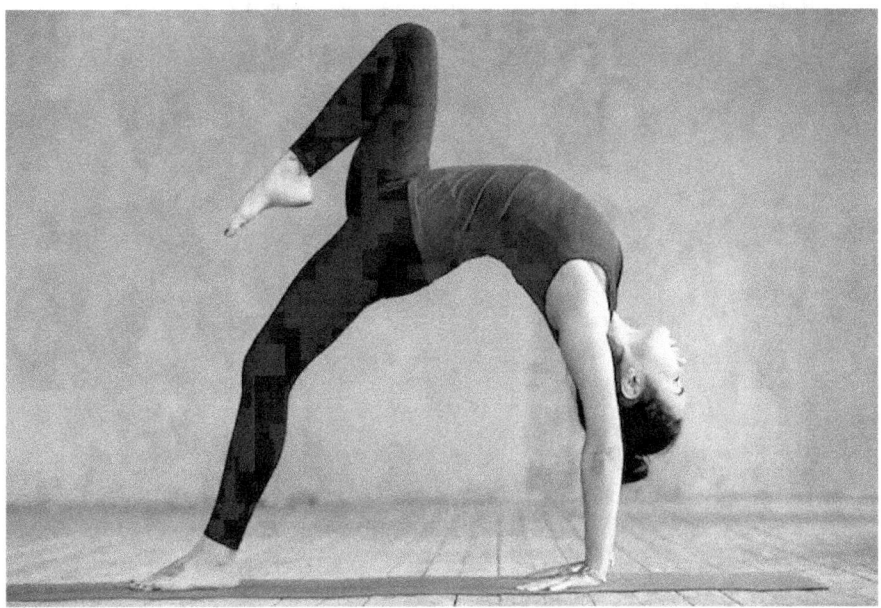

Day 2: Boat Pose and Review of Week 2

For one minute, begin in easy pose. Then, hold each of the following poses for one minute: triangle, upward dog, seated twist, pigeon, dolphin, and half wheel. Remember to perform Triangle, Seated Twist, and Pigeon poses for one minute on both the right and left sides. Proceed to the new pose for Sunday, Boat Pose, after the review, and finish as usual in Corpse Pose.

In the Boat Position

1. Sit on the ground with your legs extended in front of you to begin Boat Pose after reviewing the poses from Week 2.
2. Maintain a straight posture while packing your legs.
3. As you raise your legs off the ground and make a V with your body, lean

back slightly and maintain your arms parallel to your body for balance.
4. Maintain the stance for as long as possible while focusing on your thighs and abdominal muscles' efforts to keep you still.
5. Release, then repeat the stance as often as desired.
6. Conclude by spending a minute in corpse pose.

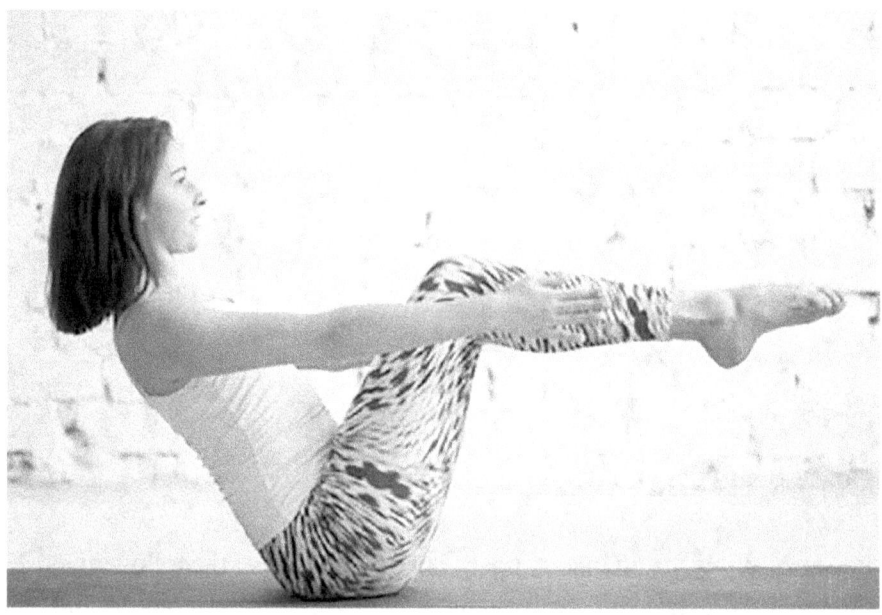

This training plan can be repeated every two weeks after the second week, or you can make up your own by combining your favorite poses.

9

Suggestions for Novices

Suggestions for Novices in Yoga

Starting a yoga practice is exhilarating. Working at your own pace and maintaining an open mind are important if you've never done this before and are unsure of what to anticipate. It's not essential to immediately become proficient in the trickiest poses and positions. Here are some pointers that will equip you with the knowledge and self-assurance you need to get going in this chapter. What's most crucial to remember is to persevere. You are making a long-term and wise decision when you commit to practicing yoga as a means of improving your health and losing weight. Neither yoga nor fitness trends are passing vogue. You'll discover that it's a way of life very quickly.

What Actions to Take

Searching for a friend is among the most crucial things you can accomplish. When you practice yoga with a partner, it becomes an enjoyable social and health activity that you look forward to. Still, yoga is incredibly effective when done alone. Try enrolling in a class that meets once a week or more if you can't find somebody to practice yoga with you. Numerous individuals who share your beliefs will show up to support you as you develop your yoga practice.

Make room in your home for yoga as another important "to do". A yoga studio furnished with a mat stack and mirrors on every wall is not necessary for this. You will benefit even if your lessons are held in a studio or gym and there is just a small area where you can stretch when you're stressed. Give equal attention to the mental and emotional aspects of yoga as the physical.

Throughout courses and on your own, you'll move and stretch a lot. Thus, set aside the time required for meditation, breathing exercises, and the use of positive imagery and thought processes. You should do yoga every day and incorporate it into your life.

Not What to Do

Keep your comparisons to other people aside. Maintaining even the most basic version of Mountain Pose can be difficult if you're new to yoga. That is acceptable. It is possible to work on that one position for a full day or even a week. You are not in competition with anyone, and there is no timeline. Stay strong and resist the urge to give in to emotions of inadequacy or insecurity by taking inspiration and motivation from others around you who have achieved more.

Refrain from going overboard. Excessive and rapid demands can quickly lead to burnout. Begin by working out for thirty or sixty minutes three times a week, and as your body becomes accustomed to the additional demands you're placing on it, gradually increase exercise frequency.

Let nothing get you down, not even negativity. Say "thank you" for their advice and carry on when well-meaning friends try to convince you that practicing yoga won't help you lose weight. Gaining better health and a smaller waist size doesn't require you to run marathons or spend hours lifting weights.

Essential Financial Commitments

Get a library constructed. Take in movies and DVDs, read books and periodicals. Acquire some CDs and read yoga blogs. You will remain informed and educated while also being inspired by these things.

Purchase a quality mat. A comfortable and engaging lesson might be achieved or not depending on your yoga mat. Don't be scared to test out a few yoga mats before making a purchase; there are plenty available. Discuss mat usage with others to learn what and why they appreciate certain mats. Get yoga clothing that fits properly, wicks away moisture, and doesn't restrict airflow.

You should wear fitted tops, shorts, and slacks to allow your body to flow naturally into your positions. Nonetheless, anything that is excessively snug will be painful.

Take out the clutter. Simplify your life by refusing processed foods that are high in fat, sodium, and sugar, as well as packaged meals and sweets. Keep away from them. Your body, mind, and soul can all be brought into balance by practicing yoga. Sloppiness will make you fall behind.

Think on what's local, seasonal, and fresh instead. At the first sign of hunger, load up on fruits and vegetables. Whether it's a fall clementine orange or a springtime batch of luscious berries, that ought to be your primary goal. Go to your local farmer's market on a regular basis.

Your energy for yoga will also come from lean protein. Seafood that is high in omegas, such as salmon and sardines, can be prepared using skinless chicken breasts, eggs, almonds, and oils that provide beneficial fats. In order to meet your protein needs as a vegetarian, you must eat alternative foods such as beans and lentils, tofu, and robust veggies like squash, eggplant, and mushrooms.

To sum up

This book will help you get the most out of your yoga practice. Maintain a positive attitude and get enthused about all the fascinating things yoga can teach you about your body and health. Exercise doesn't have to be like this. It alters your perspective on everything, including diet and weight loss, by reaching into your spirit. Be open to whichever direction this adventure takes you, both mentally and physically. Lastly, let me express my gratitude for having read my book. Please take a moment to write a review and share your opinions about the book on Amazon if you liked it. I would be really grateful for that!

www.ingramcontent.com/pod-product-compliance
Lightning Source LLC
LaVergne TN
LVHW020430080526
838202LV00055B/5116